The Uncensored [illegible]
of a Stu[illegible]

READY STEADY PUSH!

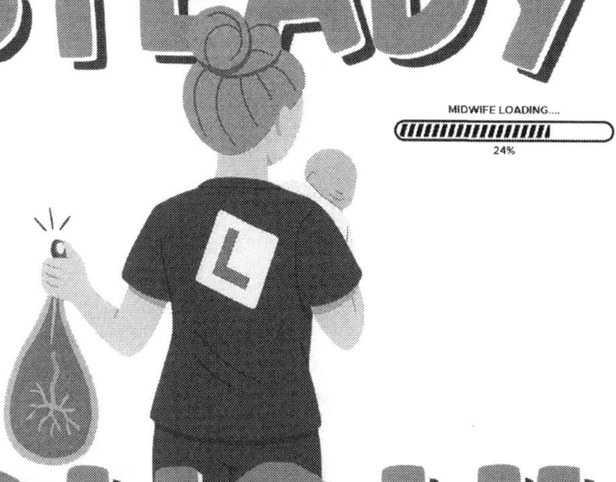

Megan Paige

Ready, Steady, Push!
The uncensored confessions of a student midwife.

ISBN: 978-1-0369-7374-2

First Edition, 2025

Independently published
Cover and interior design by Megan Paige
Printed on demand.

A NOTE BEFORE WE BEGIN/ DISCLAIMER

I am a registered midwife and bound by the Nursing and Midwifery Council (NMC) Code, which requires me to respect and protect the confidentiality of everyone in my care - as well as my colleagues.

While some stories in this book are inspired by my work, every name - apart from myself and close family and friends who have given explicit consent - is a pseudonym. Some individuals are composites; all timelines have been adjusted and identifying details have been altered or removed to ensure privacy is always upheld. Any similarities to actual people, events, or conversations - positive or negative - are purely coincidental. These accounts have been shaped for storytelling purposes and are not to be taken as a factual record.

And just to be clear, although this book offers an insight into midwifery care and guidance, it is not a medical guide. If you have any health concerns, please consult a qualified healthcare professional who can see you in person - because when it comes to birthing babies, paperbacks are best kept in the waiting room.

CONTENTS

ACKNOWLEDGMENTS

To Mum and Dad, the founding members of my all-time favourite people list. Mum, you've gotten me through life mostly backward, barefoot, and belly laughing. And honestly? It's the best. Dad, your fierce love for your people is so palpable it could probably knock over a small horse. Without you, *Ready, Steady, Push!* might still be a running joke in the group chat. It is, truly, a privilege to call you, my parents.

Al, my sister, best friend, and personal cheerleader - if I'm chaos, you're the beautiful calm that somehow still dances in the storm.

Joe, I wish you knew just how brilliant you can be. Honestly, I'd bottle it if I could.

Marsh, my non-verbal rock. I hope to one day be as carefree and present as you - though maybe not literally running outside naked and cocking your leg on Dad's shed for a wee. We'll compromise.

Grandma, absolute icon of all icons. Thank you for or never doubting me, teaching me the realest lessons and lifting my moods faster than caffeine.

Nannie and Grandad, thank you for reminding me to be unapologetically, Meg and that the sky really is the limit.

Uncle Martyn and Auntie Kim, thank you for being two of the most dedicated and inspiring people I could ever look up to. It was a long way up and I'm genuinely still a bit dizzy from the climb.

To those who are here in spirit. Grandy, I hope this book brings you a smile - we all know you loved a good laugh. Auntie Betty and Brenda, thank you for teaching me that being yourself is not just allowed, it's a bloody superpower.

To Becca and the rest of my sweep sisters. Thank you for helping me park the sadness and find joy in everything from coffee to chaos.

Liv, thank you for encouraging me to write the madness down. Life is the bubbles!

Thank you to all the patients, babies, and families who led me here. You've given me stories, lessons, and the occasional grey hair (or twenty).

And to my exceptional (and equally exhausted) colleagues and friends at my current hospital trust: the work you do is nothing short of heroic. Somehow, we survive twelve-hour (with no-wee-break) shifts, treat coffee as a food group, and turn up to do it all over again. You make me proud to be an NHS midwife every time.

PROLOGUE

At eleven, I was barely four feet tall, frizzy-haired, and convinced tie-dye could solve most of life's problems.

Eleven and a half years on the planet meant I still got on with my family and passionately played Mario Kart (on the classic Wii, of course) most days of the week.

By October 2012, I had settled into my first year of high school pretty well, and my peers seemed to accept me the same way I did them. However, there was this one guy, Ettie.

The 'popular' boys nicknamed him Sweat-ie due to his hygiene issues. I felt for him, but I gladly flew under the radar, sticking to a few quiet friends who addressed my parents as 'Meg's Mum and Dad' and evaded any sort of attention. I kept going out with my closest friends of the time, R and S, on the skateboards after school, the seven o'clock curfew was religiously respected, and I still got a huge buzz of excitement when Grandy gifted me a pound for sweets at the corner shop. Eleven marked a transitionary period of my life between the comfort of primary school perspectives and brutal teenage reality and all the feelings and changes that came with that. Nevertheless, the only thing I really had to worry about every month was saving up to top up my phone credit on my little Blackberry and who would pick me up from school. It was the calm before the storm.

Speaking of storms, in March of 2013, I'd turned twelve by then and still managed to enjoy art and geography whilst I tolerated PE and realised maths certainly wasn't for me.

Anyway, on the fifteenth of March, there was a severe weather warning for flooding in our neighbourhood. Everyone seemed to take this news as a prompt to rush to their nearest supermarket and buy toilet rolls and soup, of all things. Aside from odd shopping choices and preparing for World War Three, the school I went to attracted a lot of attention because it was built into the ground, where ground level was actually on par with the second floor of most school buildings. Clever, right?

Half a meter of rain and the place became a public swimming pool. I wonder if they had ever considered the consequences of a flash flood on a school half under ground level before they built it the way they did...

Thinking back the morning of the fifteenth of March, I tied the buckles of my recently polished, black leather shoes, completing my school morning routine. As if on cue, there was a knock on the front door. I flung it open, and both of our sheepdogs (Max and Millie, aka M&M) burst past me like I was the front door to a new world.

'Morning Meg,' S said brightly while R stood waving on the other side of the road. My dogs weren't sympathetic to his allergies.

'Bye, Mum!' I shouted up the stairs as I hauled my bag onto my back. I was still so small that the top of the rucksack smacked the back of my neck. The bottom grazed my coccyx. I looked like a walking turtle, if the turtle had a P.E. kit and undiagnosed anxiety.

'Have a good day!' boomed a voice from upstairs. As I was shoeing the dogs away, I was sure I heard my nine-year-old sister tell my six-year-old brother that he shouldn't dig his cornflakes up with his toy digger and eat them as 'it wasn't clean'. I found out later that in response, Joe forcefully pushed the digger through Al's Weetabix, to which she poured his cornflakes over his head.

Mum later banned unsupervised cereal sessions after coming down the stairs to find each dog assigned to her children, one licking the cornflakes off of Joe's forehead and the other clearing up the Weetabix from Al.

Leaving family life behind for the next eight hours, I held my bag straps with each hand and walked steadily between my two best friends.

The rain was heavy already; droplets were comparable to the size of small peas, and they fell at speed. S put up his big football umbrella, and we huddled underneath it for a while, but it was no use; the rain was getting us from any and every angle.

He ended up putting it away when a Range Rover drove through a dip in the road with momentum and sent a mini tidal wave up and over us all. My hair was drenched and slapped to my skull, and R's light grey coat turned black and sodden with water. By the time we arrived at school, puddles had already swallowed the grass, and you could only see little splinters of grass shards poking through the mucky water.

The worst revelation was finding a stream trickling down the paved steps to the main part of the school, which would never be good news. The school flooring was shining with water, and so much had collated from fellow pupils swinging around their soaked jumpers and flinging off excess rainwater. A little water seemed to have a weird effect on our peers.

Everyone seemed hyper, either shouting, fighting, or laughing; it was wild. There was also a musty smell in the air, thick with the scent of sweat and damp teenagers. Welcome to comprehensive school.

'There's so much water out there; it literally just keeps getting bigger!' S pointed out the window mid-English lesson when Mrs Aredne wasn't looking. My eyes widened as I saw the water level had risen since we arrived.

Shakespeare wasn't as captivating as he would have hoped; everyone was disengaged from his life's work and re-engaged in the current precipitation. So, the morning consisted of kids winding one another up by saying we'd all be trapped in school as the world was facing its worst case of flooding, where Noah and his arc wouldn't even be able to save us. I believed it when Johnathan the Christian seemed to approve, so I texted Mum after double English, warning her that there was a chance of us not making it home from school that day. Her response was, 'Don't be so ridiculous'. Although, in fairness, by 11.30, there was talk about closing the school as it was already causing damage to the interior of the ground floor. The water was up to my shins at break; I was so preoccupied with holding onto R and S, that I lost a few crisps to the depths en route to maths.

Maths was a mess. I hated it anyway, and for the first twenty minutes, everyone, including Mr Pary, was found to be looking out of the window, watching the water level get higher and higher. The problem was it had nowhere to go anymore; the ground level at the top of the main steps was covered in a thin film of water as the rest flowed down and filled up both the ground and the first floor.

'Excuse me, Mr Pary, but we are going to have to come in. The bottom floor is flooding, and bloody chairs are almost floating!' a flushed Mr Taylor elucidated. My Pary's class erupted in laughter as we could see the line to which the water was on Mr Taylor's trousers, above his knees. We hadn't calculated what that meant for us as he was at least two feet taller than most of us at this age.

Over the next ten minutes, our class was full of year ten students. Most of them tried to scare us until it was announced the school was closed and students were to be sent home immediately, if possible. Those stuck in the maths and science blocks were instructed to 'calmly' move to floors two or three until the fire service arrived to help.

This naturally caused an absolute uproar. Around sixty kids were cramped into a stuffy classroom, most of them screaming, 'We're all gonna die', or 'This is worse than the Titanic'. One guy was hanging out of the window, shouting for help to anyone who would listen. Another guy took it upon himself to fetch any maths textbooks he could get his hands on and throw them out of the window and into the growing sea beneath us.

'WHAT ON EARTH DO YOU THINK YOU ARE DOING?' Mr Pary bellowed as he waded through students to get to him. I'd never seen him so angry before.

'They reckon you need to make it lighter, Sir, so we prolong sinking,' he said confidently as he dropped another 'fundamental maths' textbook to its peril.

'We are in a school, not a boat in the middle of the Atlantic, Porter!' Mr Pary snatched the remaining books from his grasp.

'At least I'm being productive,' Adam Porter shrugged, mid-textbook toss. 'Unlike *her*,' he pointed at a girl sobbing into her Nokia, asking her mum to buy more eyelashes because the 'flood drowned them.'

After a while of flying textbooks and wailing teenagers, I started to feel really agitated. The number of people in the room enclosed me, and I knew I had nowhere to go, a bit like the rain. I couldn't seem to cope well with lots of voices at different volumes at the same time but at different rates. Add no replies from either of my parents, and the tears started to roll steadily down my face.

'Meg, what are you doing? We don't need any more water added to this place!' Tommy said with a sympathetic smile and a hand on my back. Tommy was one of the quiet boys in my class, a little taller than me with a stocky build. He usually kept himself to himself, so I couldn't say I knew more than that. Even still, I was so overstimulated by the raucous environment that I heard what he said, but my brain couldn't listen.

'You know I'm a champion diver when I'm not here, right?' He said proudly with his shoulders back and chest out like a proud peacock.

'What do you mean?' I asked through a blocked nose.

'I competed in a few diving competitions before coming here,' he said proudly. 'Look, I'll help you out of here, along with a few of them,' he indicated at a group of boys behind him. I looked at him, confused. Was this a joke? Before I concluded, I observed him as he edged his way to the window, used the table as a step and kneeled on the windowsill. I looked behind me and scanned the room for the teachers. I found Mr Pary consoling a boy who was having a panic attack and Mr Taylor, who was furious, on the phone on the other side of the room. I turned back to Tommy, and he gestured for us to come over with a wide smile spread across his face. The group of boys and I toddled after him. We all peered out the window to find the water level was up to the point between the first and second floors.

'Christ alive!' Jay took the words out of my mouth and frowned at the depths below.

'There's a decent amount of water for sure,' Tommy enthusiastically confirmed the obvious. 'Watch this, boys' he turned to the water and then back again, 'And girl,' and winked at me. I felt my stomach flip. He extended his arms in front of him, pushed off the windowsill, and disappeared into the water. My stomach flipped again.

He took an age to come back up, long enough for the boys and me to exchange looks of, 'When should we start to worry?'

'There he is!' one of the boys cried and pointed out. We all looked out and saw a head bobbing in the water.

'It's fine!' Tommy spluttered as he swiped his hair out of his face. 'Oi Aaron, chuck us your bag, mate!' Aaron did as instructed and lowered his black sports bag over to Tommy, who swam to the top of the steps and threw his bag onto a piece of not-so-flooded ground. He then broke into a little front crawl and came back to the building. Aaron slowly sank into the water with Tommy as support and swam to the drier ground, picked up his bag and shouted words of encouragement for the rest of us.

'Come on, then, Meg,' Tommy said, extending his arm and offering his hand for support. I stood overlooking the water, contemplating what was worse: the loud and busy classroom or treading water in the middle of my school day.

'Better in here than in there,' Tommy nodded towards the classroom as if he read my mind. I moved my hand up to my forehead, then down, and tapped each shoulder, praying this wasn't the stupidest idea I'd ever committed to. I'd love to say I hesitated on my next move. That I considered the consequences. But instead, I made direct eye contact with a year ten boy who'd just compared the situation to 'the end of the world' and leapt. I felt the cold water hit me and flailed my arms around. Tommy's hands under my arms held me up. I eventually bobbed to the top of the water.

'Ugh,' I panted, holding onto the wall with my right hand, and wiped my eyes with my left one. I was actually gripped to the side of my school, in deep, cold water, in my uniform.

'See, there you go,' Tommy reassured me. 'Remember, I'm a champion diver!' He looked so calm and collected. Meanwhile, under the water, my legs were peddling as fast as I could, and I was trying to avoid taking in any more gulps of muddy water.

'You go, and I'll follow you, Meg,' Tommy nudged me as I broke into a little breaststroke and swam my way to dry (ish) land.

When I got there, I looked back towards the building and spotted R and S in the third-floor window, jaws on the floor. They couldn't believe that Meg 'never took a risk' Paige had made her great escape. I waved at them and shouted,

'I got saved by Tommy!' I pointed at him, making his way back steadily to get someone else's bag. 'He's a champion diver, you know!' I said through the cheesiest smile. I still remember Mum's confusion when I arrived home sopping wet and covered top to toe in mud. It was when I proceeded to tell her proudly that I had jumped out of the window from the second floor that she almost fainted.

'What on earth did you just say?' Mum looked alarmed. I gave her the much-needed context to the story, and she calmed down once she'd ruled out if I was either hurt, hypothermic or needing additional psychological help.

'Only you can say you swam home from school, Meg,' she shook her head after I told her about Tommy and his debut. 'You always manage to be part of something funny or a little bit pear-shaped, I have to say,' she smiled as I peeled off my soggy uniform and gave it to her to wash. 'Walking through chaos again, Meg?' Dad asked, raising his eyebrows as I dripped mud onto the kitchen floor.

'We'll have to call you Walking Chaos,' Mum laughed. And there it was. The moment I became a walking punchline, with soggy socks and a knock off diving qualification.

INTRODUCTION

Fast forward eleven years, and a lot has happened since I jumped out of my first window. My parents were right; even from a young age, I always seemed to be a part of something comedically chaotic.

Whether that was something going wrong; like when I took Mum's bike out with the boys, they rode through the shallow brook with no problems; I tried to catch up, wedged the tyre between two rocks and flew off it into the mud mound on the other side. Having R and S unstick teenage me from a mudslide wasn't on my bucket list, it has to be said.

Or whether it was something going right even, such as showing my sister how to blow out a candle. I swept the hair out of the way, etc. (safety first), only to find I blew the candle out so effectively that the wax rebounded onto my face, burnt my lip and lower nose, I looked like I had some sort of virus for weeks. But at least I had a little wax sculpture of my features as a reminder to Al and me of what not to do. Whatever it was, there was some sort of complication. However, life, of course, is not always laughs and rainbows; quite often, its cries and rainclouds. But the experiences, good and not so good, ultimately shape who we are. I've learned that shadows will always hide behind the sunshine, but embracing the humorous side of most things has been the best way to manage; for me, that's for sure.

I'm a practising midwife now, but wow, the story of getting here, being here, and projecting more of my life here is one to get comfortable and your popcorn out for. Starting from the flood of 2013 to qualifying in 2022 as a midwife, we've got a fair few chapters to negotiate.

From elation to total devastation, oppressed to conquered, this is what this book is all about, capturing some of the best, the worst and the damn right craziness of a lifetime of twenty-four years and counting. Welcome to *Ready, Steady, Push!* where the plan is never the plan, and somehow, that's always been the point.

PART 1

Growing Up

CHAPTER

One

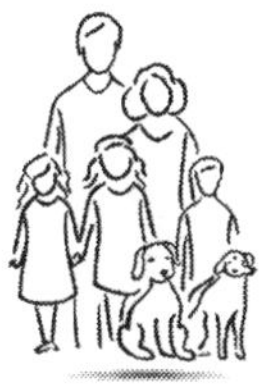

MASSIVE SLUG

A year after the flood, I exuded thirteen years of life experience. I was only just leaning into my teenage self where I gradually became more conscious of my body as it altered. My frizzy hair and awkward way of carrying my square shape miraculously didn't faze me. Although, the unwelcome visits from the hormone family came bearing gifts of spots so enraged they looked as though they were trying to push through my skin at every given chance. But I didn't really care too much. I still lived in a blissful place of accepting myself for who I was. Maybe I could have given my latter teenage years a few tips. But that's for another time.

My Saturdays were typically still marked as free, so I'd usually go shopping with Mum or spend my time outside with R and S. However, reflecting on a particular Saturday, mid-April I couldn't do either of those tasks due to awful weather. Thankfully, the rainwater didn't reach a level where I needed to call on Tommy like the previous year. Nevertheless, with R and S taking cover from the rain in their respective homes and Mum sorting a few things out in ours, I gave into that burning teenage need for infinite sleep and slept in until at least eleven o'clock. Then I sat in bed and watched *The Lion King*. My life was as simple as these sentences sound. It was a great time to be alive.

'Meg! Let me in!' Al shouted from outside my bedroom door. She was ten now and had undoubtedly found her voice.

'Come in,' I said, pausing where Mufasa had just died. Immediately, Al burst through the door.

'Sam's off again!' Al burst in, buzzing with gossip about our fifteen-year-old next-door neighbour totally ignoring the fact I was mid-mourning Mufasa.

'Who's he arguing with?' I placed my bets on it being Sam's Mum, Jen.

'Jen!' Boom. They argued most days, but more often than not, it got quite cataclysmic between them. My bedroom was adjacent to Sam's, so I could hear a lot without even trying. Al's room, however, was next to mine but sandwiched between my room and our parents, therefore, protected from the Smiths. Like most families, the Smiths endured their utmost dramatic stuff after school. Despite Al and I listening intently for our entertainment, the things we heard over the years sure made you feel lucky you weren't on the other side of the wall.

'Twat bag!!' Sam's voice boomed. We gasped like he'd just murdered his Nan. Even Al, who once told off a dinner lady for forgetting her salad cream, looked scandalised.

'You little tramp, you do nothing for me or this family,' Jen retorted. I grimaced at her insult. 'I found a half-eaten chicken drumstick in your pillowcase yesterday; it's disgusting,' Jen shouted. *A chicken drumstick*. I'm sorry but what kind of poultry-based goblin keeps a half-eaten carcass as a security blanket? For two kids who still thought 'pull my finger' was top-tier comedy, this was next-level. I was smacking my wardrobe as I creased with laughter, and Al giggled her way to a red face. Back then, I didn't have the capacity to think sincerely about it and consider how hostile that environment was and how detrimental it was to all living in it.

'You're a massive slag; leave me alone,' Sam bellowed.

'Did he just call his mum the 's' word Meg?' Al turned to me, concerned.

'Yep,' I verified what she had just heard.

'Meg, can I come in?' A little voice spoke. Al and I turned from the conjoining wall to face my bedroom door.

'Are you alright, Joe?' I asked as I opened the door. He was only seven and crying in Fireman Sam pyjamas.

'What's the matter?' I said as I hugged his little body.

'Sam called his Mum a massive slug!' Joe exclaimed.

'Actually, he said -,'Al went to say and stopped as I shook my head vigorously at her.

'It's not very nice, is it?' I said, desperately trying to think of a way around this. 'Don't worry, though. Families argue, and they will sort it out,' I tried to reassure him, but as if on cue, Jen shouted 'little prick' back to him. Excellent.

'Is it because she looks like a slug?' Joe asked as he swapped his upset for curiosity.

'Pahaha,' Al was set off again, and I couldn't help but let out a little laughter, too.

'She does look like one sometimes,' Joe said in deep introspection.

'Even if she does resemble a slug, he shouldn't say it because it is unkind, right?' I hoped to end his train of thought.

'Fucking wanker bitch!' Sam screamed. Both Al and my eyes shot wide open.

'Meg, what's a wanker bitch?' Joe asked, wide-eyed and innocent in his Fireman Sam pyjamas. Brilliant. Just what I needed: a crash course in creative swearing, primary school edition.

'Just... don't say that at school, yeah?' I said weakly. He nodded and then went on to try to write it in play dough with a plastic spoon.

CHAPTER
Two

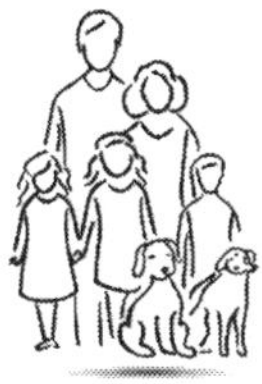

THE 800-METRE STRIP

The months rolled by, and the end of year eight was on the horizon. A lot had happened in ten months; R started to grow a stray collection of dark hair on his chin, which he reported getting congratulations from his dad. He was chuffed about it as his dad was in the army and known for not being easily pleased, so naturally, R spent much time nurturing his five sacred hairs. Meanwhile, S's voice was still a few octaves higher than R's, and he struggled with that concept a little, especially when other friends couldn't tell whether it was S or me talking to them.

As for me, my body had a couple of malfunctions whereby I sprouted little teepees for boobs overnight, and my vagina started to cry blood every month. I couldn't believe my luck to have to deal with it twelve times a year. Still, it wasn't until Mum told me that we *all* have to deal with it twelve times a year, and it wasn't a lucky dip for how many times each person menstruates that I accepted it's normality. Either way, with high notes, budding teepees and sprouting beards, the three of us were still as good friends as we had ever been.

'Meg, you need to hurry up!' R shouted as he sprinted ahead to complete his second lap of the 800-metre track before I'd even done my first. Running was never for me. My boobs flopped East and West, my belly jiggled North and South, and I was essentially a human compass with no direction. Plus, the sweltering heat of June, in the field with no shade, in a sticky school polo shirt, was not the one.

'Meg, watch out!' S whispered harshly between breaths as he jogged past me. I turned around to see our PE teacher, Miss Davies, approaching. Damn. As I picked up my feet to resume, I cupped my boobs with my hands and tried to stop them from flailing around. It worked for a few moments, but I had to stop again. My chest was tight, and I was thirsty enough to drain the Serengeti and still ask for squash.

'You can do better than that, Megan,' Miss Davies said on her arrival. She was about six feet tall, had blonde hair in a perfect ponytail, and it swished when she ran. To top it off, she didn't have one ounce of sweat on her skin. On the contrary, my skin was bright red, sweat escaped every pore. As for the rest of me, my boobs were taking a beating like two hamsters in a knock-off boxing ring, cheap gloves, no forgiveness. As for my inner thighs, they were hosting a slip-

and-slide for sweat. *Sweaty inner thighs.* It was at that moment I was confirmed to be an actual mess.

'I can't do this, Miss,' I plucked at my slightly damp leggings.

'You can, it's mind over matter, yes?' She sternly said as she got a bottle of water from her rucksack for me. 'Jog alongside me for a moment,' she encouraged me. It wasn't that the exercise was too much (it was), but it was also the sweat making me feel uncomfortable, to say the least. I tried to ignore it whilst we jogged for a little while, but when I felt a few big droplets of sweat descending down my back and feeling the two collide at the base of my spine, that was my limit. I felt a wave of stress, and the most uncomfortable feeling arrived.

'I can't do this anymore,' I declared and ran impulsively towards the shade.

'Megan, come back here, please!' Miss Davies shouted as she veered off the course to follow me

'Everybody carry on, I will be two minutes!' She bellowed to her little tribe of year eights.

'Megan! Where are you going?' I heard her but couldn't take anything in. All that was on my mind was that I needed to get those damp leggings off me as they were hurting my skin (I perceived the feeling as pain, at least).

'What's going on?' She caught up with me as I was midway putting my arms down my leggings, extending them in front of me to create space between them and my legs. 'I need you to return to the group now, please,' she sighed as if I was her fifty-first inconvenience that day (I probably was her 151st). The fusion of skin and leggings got too much so I instinctively yanked those leggings off like they were on fire, launched them into the nearest tree, and stood there in neon pink pants like a damp, raging fairy. I can confirm my pale bum cheeks were poking out of my bright pink Primark pants, in the middle of a field, in front of all of my peers, during my school day. I seemed to go into a hyper-focused mode and had gained awareness of my own body parts; it felt like I could feel every cell in my arms, legs, ankles even. Was it even possible to feel claustrophobic inside of your own limbs?

I could hear the muffled people's voices in the distance, the rustling leaves from the tree above, and small insects beating their wings through the thick summer air around me.

'Come with me, Meg,' a different voice said before me. I looked up and was relieved to see a familiar face. It was Lyssa, a girl from my year. I had no idea how much time had passed, though I realised she wasn't in my PE class. Nevertheless, her kind eyes were fixed upon mine, and her long, brown hair tumbled before her face. Lucky for me, Lyssa was actually a good friend of mine and she only lived a few streets away. We would often share a bag of chips from the Chinese on a Friday night while her mum let us watch Big Brother. Those were the days.

'Come on,' she offered me her hand. I locked my hand into hers and silently got up, and she covered me with a grey frayed towel. Where did she get a towel from? I certainly hadn't seen Miss Davies whip one out from her rucksack. I looked around and scouted for my classmates, but no one was on the field either. Where were R and S?

'Miss Davies sent them the long way around to the changing rooms, so they didn't go past you,' Lyssa clocked onto my confusion. 'She's alright once she stops shouting,' Lyssa shrugged. 'And don't worry, we've all had a public pants moment.'

'Have we though?' I muttered.

'Well... I peed on my mum's new rug last week when I laughed too hard.'

'I haven't wet myself, Lyssa!' I exclaimed as I felt my cheeks flush with embarrassment.

'Oh, sorry, I just thought,' she stopped herself as I started to cry. Instead, she put her arm around me and simultaneously released the towel from her grasp. It dropped from my waist and exposed my knickers once again. Brilliant. We both giggled, and eventually, I pulled the thinning towel back up and we headed for the changing rooms.

I spent the rest of the day feeling like that tired old towel, slightly damp, a bit frayed, and barely holding it together. I spent the whole of history reflecting on the events of PE rather than World War Two and worried about what all of that meant. When I asked R and S, R said it wasn't a big deal, and S said it sounded like something his brother would do; he was five. In all fairness, it was Miss Davies who mentioned the word 'autistic' to my parents at parent's evening. Still, considering grades were fine, and my social appearance was also apparently fine, it was deemed something I would 'grow out of', like sensory overload was just a weird hobby. Although, being thirteen and feeling out of place in the world because it felt like you were the only one where wearing leggings made you feel like I was being slow-roasted alive, it was only you who cried for weeks because your parents gave your next-door neighbours the front door and you were so distraught with the change your parents had to re-buy it off them when they gave it to them for free in the first place; it was only you that couldn't eat pizza with toppings on because there was no consistency with every bite. But without a name for it, it just felt like I was the only one who couldn't handle the world without falling apart.

Spoiler alert: you don't grow out of being neurodivergent. You just get better at hiding it. Preferably with your leggings on.

CHAPTER *Three*

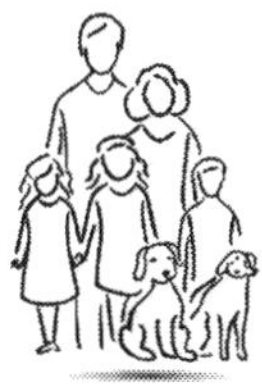

END OF AN ERA

July of 2014 was the end of Year Eight and the abrupt end of Llantarnam Comprehensive School. We spent the last few months signing any and every petition, fighting hard for the school to remain open; ultimately, the government had already decided. We felt they allowed us to vote, which gave us a false sense of thinking it mattered. Democracy, Welsh comprehensive school edition. By the end of July, they released a statement declaring they wanted its 'flat land' to build on. However, I couldn't help but wonder how they seemed to have forgotten how fifty percent of the school was submerged underwater during the floods of 2013. Tommy's outdoor diving debut sprang to mind once again. Speaking of Tommy, he swapped diving for open-water swimming, which shocked everyone, except me. The boy practically lived amphibiously.

'What am I actually going to do, Mum?' I asked as I watched her flip the toast over for the third time one Sunday morning.

'You've got two options,' she said, still armed with a butter knife. Nothing says negotiation like a Mum holding cutlery. 'Either go with your friends and relocate to the new school, or we see if we can get you into Croeswen,' She hovered by the grill, anticipating my response to a change of any kind.

'I don't want to go to either,' I muttered. Mum's face dropped like she'd just driven a car made of hope straight into a brick wall of reality.

'Llant is closed, Meg,' she said as she noticed the toaster smoking slightly. 'Ahh, God,' she grimaced as she transferred the steaming toast to the plates on the kitchen counter. 'Al. Joe. FOOD!' she shouted to the ascending stairs. I put my fingers in my ears and awaited their arrival.

Al arrived first. She was eleven now and looked about six in her Scooby-Do pyjamas. She clambered onto her breakfast stool beside me and poked my hip.

'Mum, can I have jam, please?' Al asked as she swept her blonde hair out of her face. Mum seemed to be some sort of psychic with us and was unscrewing the lid of the jam before we'd even asked for it.

'I like raspberry jam, Mum,' Al said skeptically as she investigated the jam before her.

'Sorry, Al. It's Meg who likes the strawberries, isn't it?' Mum said as she switched the jams around. Al looked like someone had just demoted her from 'main character' to 'supporting role'. Like most middle children, she will tell you that 'middle child syndrome' is a very real phenomenon that she has to live with for her entire existence. I couldn't relate; I once signed a card to my parents for Valentine's Day that I had made at school with 'Love, your eldest and bestest kid'... Anyway, jam or no jam, Joe was nowhere to be seen. In the end, Mum had to go and physically get him from upstairs, as he was too engrossed in building a Lego spaceship. Breakfast was, therefore, an inconvenience in his day, and he sat with his arms crossed in frozen frustration until Mum put some Nutella on his toast. He eventually defrosted and smiled to himself as he ate it. It was the little things.

'Meg, Meg, can we sleep over Grandma's? She said all of us could when school was finished,' Al turned to me with excitement plastered on her face. 'Joe, are you coming?' Al waved her hand at him.

'Yeah!' He punched the air in excitement, launching a globule of Nutella into the air. It hit the wall with a splat and stuck there like a sugary omen.

'Yes, yes, this will be so much fun!' I caught a glimpse of their excitement and forgot about my school placement for a second.

'Right, Meg. Can you walk and talk for a minute while I hang the washing outside?' Mum asked as she saw my face fall again. I nodded and followed her to the garden.

I stepped outside, and I could feel the warmth of the pavement through my socks; the summer sun had warmed it gently throughout the morning, and the air already looked hazy. Millie was basking in the heat at the top of the garden;

meanwhile, Max, who hated most things, including the sun, was snoozing in his kennel. We were lucky to have a big garden and lots in it; a little climbing frame, a trampoline, toys, Joe's little car and even a football goal for Al. However, a few years ago, Mum divided the garden, half for kids, half for dogs, after I flew down the slide and crash-landed in a pile of dog poo. Joe cried because he wasn't allowed to make mud pies with it. Al tried to solve the crime by following both dogs around, analysing their butts like a forensic vet. Mum spent the next three weeks bleaching my clothes, my shoes, and probably me. Therefore, strategic segregation was introduced, and we haven't had one of those events for a few years now.

Anyway, back to the present day, I decided to venture to the other side of the fence and sat with Millie as we often ended up doing. She wagged her tail lazily when I smoothed her sun-kissed fur. I watched as Mum pulled down the reluctant washing line. I looked down at Millie and returned to find four tops and a dress already on the line. She was like a machine. The next time I looked up, she'd have probably finished another load and would need to bring them back off again.

'I was chatting with Dad, and we think we should try and get you into Croeswen,' she opened the conversation once more. 'Both your cousins go there, and it has much better reports than the other school you'd be merging with,' she said as she flung a pair of Dad's boxers over the line.

'But I don't know anyone there,' my voice cracked like it had a secret it wasn't ready to spill. Millie, the dog, immediately sensed doom and tried to wedge her head into my lap like a therapy cushion with paws.

'Lots of people start new schools, Meg; you will make new friends and keep in touch with your old ones, too, that doesn't have to change,' Mum said with a look of sympathy which seemed to trigger my full-on tears. 'Change can sometimes be a good thing; you've always got to give it time,' she said gently as she hugged me. 'Give it six weeks and look at where you are compared to where you started, and you'll be amazed at the difference.' I took it literally as six weeks, and my life would be back to normal, which wasn't quite what Mum was going for, but it worked at that moment. 'Plus, I've spoken to R and S's parents, and they are on board for trying to get the three of you in together.' That was enough for me as R and S meant the world, so I relaxed and spent the next hour reading one of the Harry Potter books and stroking the dog. I watched as Al launched footballs at the house as it was the only thing that could pass back to her, Joe disappeared to his room, and Mum whizzed around on the phone, cleaning, back on the phone. I wondered how she did it.

Over the next few weeks, R's Dad, S's parents, and I collaborated to appeal for us all to have space in Croeswen. To all of our surprise, they won. They managed to win them over, with thirty pupils in every form except for two, which had twenty-eight and twenty-nine, giving enough clauses for us to fill the spaces. R and S were stoked. I... was less stoked. It didn't just feel like the school was closing. It felt like someone had dismantled the stage mid-performance, and I was left whispering my lines to an empty audience. But six weeks, Mum said. Six weeks, and I'd feel different. And if not? Well, worst case, Tommy could teach me how to dive out of that one too.

CHAPTER

Four

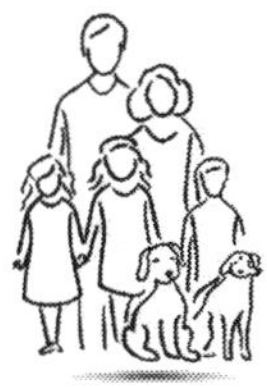

WELCOME TO TEENAGE HELL

Monday, the first of September 2014. New day. New week. New uniform. New pit in my stomach. Same old me, just repackaged in itchy tights and blind panic. The day had finally arrived, and I woke with a lump already lodged in the back of my throat.

Thanks to adrenaline, I shot out of bed at 07:01 and tried to convince myself it would all be fine. *All fine*. I watched myself in the mirror, taking a few exaggerated breaths. I was already on edge, my new shirt felt like cardboard, the tag on my tights itched my back, and just to top it all off, I looked down at my jumper and saw the new school emblem. That was it. The final straw. Mum ended up on the floor with her arms wrapped around me as I cried in a ball, trying desperately to remove myself from the world. Funnily enough, it didn't work. And when I finally opened my eyes and squinted over her shoulder at the clock on the wall, the emblem was still there, and it was time to leave. Balls.

The car journey was much better once R and S joined. I felt so lucky to have them. R, always the laid-back one, reminded us of the move being only temporary as with most things in life. S, ever the perfectionist, kept licking his fingers and plastering his fringe back into place. But within seconds, a few strands would flop sadly forward again. I never thought I'd have more in common with S's hair than my peers at that point - but there I was. Wilted and needing reviving, and I hadn't even clapped eyes on the place I'd be spending the next three years of my life. Eventually, after a relentless stream of thoughts, we pulled up to the school gates.

'Thanks, Mrs H,' R smiled as he jumped out and looked around. S followed, using the car window as a mirror in one last attempt to salvage his fringe. I lingered. Mum and I exchanged a look - one of those rare, silent ones that spoke much louder than words. If she'd said anything nice, I'd have folded completely. So, neither of us said a word. A true miracle. I climbed out, hastily re-tucking my jumper into my skirt, making sure there was nothing anyone could use to call me out. I just wanted to remain quiet - strategically invisible.

'Ready?' R asked, gesturing toward the building. I took in a sharp breath and followed R and S into the unknown.

As the three of us joined the stream of students heading in, a group of girls scurried past. A separate gang of boys hurled water bottles at them. That ended badly for one lad who soaked a girl's trousers. She kneed him square in the balls and promised that if he tried again, she'd crush them to dust. Brutal, yet fair. The school felt massive, probably because we didn't have a clue where anything was. Everything seemed dark and unfamiliar. I started breathing faster. Mum's six-week rule popped into my head, and I clung to it like a life raft.

Thankfully, I'd re-regulated by the time we reached reception, where a lovely woman named Janice greeted us from behind a high wooden desk. She looked to be in her sixties, with long grey hair pinned neatly to the sides of her kind, warm face. She radiated hug energy, the kind of woman who smelled like Polo mints and backup tissues. We all liked Janice instantly. She handed us planners and timetables and explained our form groups, two together, one solo. R and I had identical timetables, which left S on his own.

I felt equal parts relieved and guilty, but S didn't seem fussed. If anything, both he and R looked relieved that they wouldn't be dealing with my third emotional meltdown of the morning. Fair enough. By nine o'clock, things were falling into place. Janice had shown us which toilets were blocked, which vending machines only worked with a well-placed kick, and which teachers not to mess with. We liked Janice even more. By eleven o'clock, I'd met my form tutor, Mr Arnold, R had eaten three apples between form and RE and looked like he might start photosynthesising. And I was already so overstimulated I needed a dark corner, and it wasn't even midday.

Considering how fixated my teenage brain had been on all the negatives, the rest of that first week actually went pretty well. We didn't get hopelessly lost, S was doing fine in his form, and R and I had settled into ours too. I even made a new friend, Nina. She lived five minutes from school with her mum, her nan, and their fourteen-year-old Jack Russell, Johno. Jack Russells seemed to live forever. My auntie's dog, Jasper, made it to nineteen. Lisa from across the road had one too, he was fifteen last time I asked, and he'd already outlived her second marriage. Anyway, Nina, her mum, nan, and Johno were all lovely, and they made the transition feel far less grim. R and S liked her too, so soon, three became four. For the first time in nearly fourteen years, I wasn't outnumbered. I finally had a girl I could call my friend. I was chuffed.

One drizzly breaktime, as we huddled under the science block to escape the sideways rain, Nina nudged me and whispered,

'R's so fit, don't you think?' I laughed, assuming she was joking. R was basically my brother. But when I turned, her cheeks were bright red.

'What?' she grinned. 'He's funny... and honestly, really cute when he smiles,' she said in a tone I'd not heard before. I smiled back, encouraging her as I also thought the world of him. After that, I started to notice the signs - how she blushed when he cracked a joke, how she subtly smoothed her hair when he walked past. I realised Nina and I shared love for R in very different ways. It was sweet and simple. Until the sweet turned sour, and the simple became anything but.

LESSON 1: WELSH, WITH MRS MICHAELS

Everyone in my Welsh class seemed to be feral, so the only good thing about that class was sitting next to Nina. Until the day I found her crying.

'Nina, you can tell me what's wrong. You know that,' I whispered gently.

'No, I can't,' she snuffled. 'Not anymore.' That *anymore* made my stomach twist.

'Have I done something?' I asked, heart thumping.

'You know how much I liked R,' she said as tears rolled down her face.

'Yeah, of course. What's happened?' I asked. I'd genuinely rooted for them. R and S were like brothers to me.

'As if you didn't know,' Nina snapped. 'I don't ever want to see you again, Megan.'

That hit like a punch to the chest. My eyes filled instantly.

'And what are you two whispering about that's more important than my class?' Mrs Michaels called out, drawing everyone's attention. Thanks a bunch, Miss.

'Meg slept with R!' Callum bellowed like he'd just read the morning headlines. 'She's a slag for doing that to Nina!' Slag. Me. I hadn't even looked at a boy, let alone slept near one, unless you count sharing bunk beds with a guy called Harry, aged six, and even then, I was top bunk with a guard rail.

'Oh my God, who would even go near her?' Christian laughed. 'She's well ugly. Nothing like Nina!' The classroom erupted. Some laughed. Some jeered. Mrs Michaels tried to hush them, but it was useless.

'You're not even denying it,' Tristan spat as if my silence was a confession. 'You're actually nasty.' Without thinking, I shoved my books into my bag with shaking hands.

'I didn't do it!' I said, barely above a whisper. 'I'd never do that to you, Nina!' But she was already gone. And so was I.

Unsurprisingly, that was the last thing I said out loud for a long time. To this day, I'm not sure who actually started the rumour. Maybe Callum made it up for laughs. Maybe Nina needed a villain. Either way, the rumour spread like wildfire, and I couldn't trust anyone. Even Benny from French and Rhys from Maths, boys who didn't usually get involved in drama, kept their distance. Their silence stung, but not like R and S's did. R said he knew it wasn't true but thought we needed space. *Space?* I was the one being torn to shreds. He corrected the rumour, to save himself, but refused to hang out with me anymore, not even outside school. As for S? He didn't want the heat of association either. So, he ignored me completely. I was gutted. I lost my best friends, my new friend and myself all in one week. Welcome to teenage hell.

CHAPTER
Five

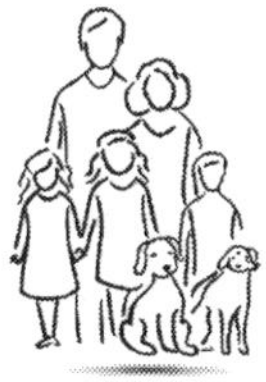

THE AFTERMATH

The weeks rolled on, and the group of four was no more; Nina found herself in love with another guy by January, and after all the trouble she threw my way, I had decided I wasn't missing much. As for R and S, I felt it hit me much harder when they went diving head-first into a new friendship pool. To be fair to them, they did well, they were a nice group of boys, and I was merely gutted that I wasn't part of it. I even tried to reach out to Tommy in the hope that because he was in a different school, he wouldn't know anything, but my texts were never returned.

So, the new year may have brought Nina a new boyfriend and R and S a new group, but for me, I had a different kind of friendship quartet going on; Sadness, Fear, Loneliness and

Anxiety. None of them were good listeners. But they always turned up. Uninvited, obviously. They fed off each other the more I gave in to them too which ultimately made them the most toxic and dangerous friends I'd made to date. Quite frankly, they caused a right flipping mess.

No thanks to my new friendship group, I became withdrawn, and every time Mum asked me what was wrong, I seemed to automatically snap and shout, which caused an argument between us. It all fell to shit, really, like my life had been tidily stacked, then kicked over by a tantruming toddler with brass knuckles. I felt feelings of desperate sadness unlike any I had felt before. Dad and I had been growing more and more distant lately too. We'd barely exchanged more than a few sharp words since the school move.

My perspective of the world had crumbled from a fairly trusting place to one of deception and fear. They always said teenagers felt emotions to the highest degree, and once again this is what made it all so destructive. I went from believing I was a person deserving of good things to thinking I was not in a matter of months. For five out of seven days a week I was told I was 'ugly' or fat' or 'a waste of space', by multiple different people, and for me, the empirical evidence was conclusive. I was convinced of the words they had spoken and was so consumed by the negative that the rare positive fell like a grain of sugar in a cup of tea, unnoticed and ineffective.

'WHAT!' I slammed my fist down onto my desk after hearing Mum call my name for the third time outside of my bedroom door.

'Come on, Meg, this isn't you! Being a teenager is hard; changing schools is hard-'

'If you hadn't made me move to that stupid school, I wouldn't be so miserable would I!' I ripped my school tie off as I shouted back, feeling the pent-up anger take over my body. 'I literally HATE everything about it, Mum! The people call me anything but my name, the teachers don't even care to know my name, EVERYTHING IS JUST AWFUL!' I roared unnecessarily. I felt guilty when I looked up to face Mum and watched a tear pave its way down her face. It wasn't her fault any more than it was mine. Deep down, I knew that, but I was blinded by hurt and ignited by anger.

A few hours later, I put on a fluffy jumper, picked up a chocolate bar from the corner shop, and headed to the kitchen to give it to Mum as an apology. However, she wasn't there. Instead, Dad was sitting at the table.

'She's had enough, Meg. And honestly, so have I,' he looked up sadly from the table. 'You push everyone away and then act surprised when they don't come back.' He brushed past me which knocked the chocolate bar out of my hands. It broke as it hit the floor and slammed the front door behind him. My chest was on fire. I slapped my hand flat over my heart like I could press the pain down, shut it up. I was gasping, dizzy, convinced this was it, death by feelings. I gasped for breath and ran around the kitchen thinking that this was how it felt to have a heart attack and that I was going to die before I'd even got to the good bit, like prom, or finally growing boobs. Turns out I didn't die, but I spent the next few hours in the corner of my room contemplating everything. Gladly, my phone distracted me and started to ring at about two hours in. It was Grandma.

CHAPTER
Six

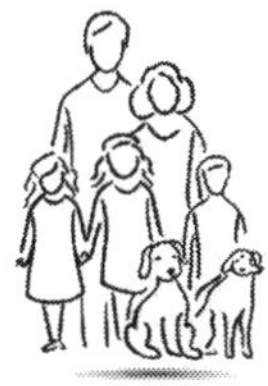

GRANDMA

'Hello?' I tried to sound as normal as I possibly could.

'Hello love, it's Grandma, how are you doing?' The kindest voice from the kindest person hit my ears. So naturally, I burst into tears.

'I don't know,' I took a breath, 'what-to-do-anymore-Grandma,' my words were almost robotic.

'Come to my place and tell me all about it,' she said calmly. Nothing phased Grandma; it was one of the many things that made her the most brilliant human I know. When we lost Grandy in the early half of last year, it undoubtedly shattered us all, yet she always reminded us of any ounce of light in mere darkness. She told us it would always be there if we knew to look hard enough. She was merely incredible.

As soon as Grandma hung up, I chucked my thin, black school rain jacket on and headed downstairs. I caught sight of myself in the mirror as I tugged to get my feet in my shoes. I wasn't really sure as to who was looking back at me. My mousy brown hair was scraped in a bun; my face was expressionless. A pair of icy blue eyes stared back at me, swollen from emotion, yet they looked vacant now where only the shadows of my sadness remained. I swiped my bunch of keys and felt the horn of the little unicorn key ring press against my palm. I reflected on a distant memory of R giving it to me after he won it on a two-pence machine years ago. I admired the little guy for a moment, but as I put the keys in the door, he dropped to the floor, and his head popped clean off. If that wasn't the most on-brand metaphor for my life at that point, I don't know what was. I picked up the pieces of him as, yet another warm memory frosted over.

Following a brisk five-minute walk, I had arrived at Grandma's house. One of the perks of having Grandma? She was literally around the corner. She lived at number ninety-eight, right on the end of the street. Her house was ivory white and had a huge garden to which I had felt fantastic memories flood through the moment I saw it. I think my conscious memories of chaos may have originated there. For example, a few years back, we spent a beautiful summer's day at number ninety-eight, but amongst all the fun, we lost Joe to the bush and found him three hours later in a little nook, happy as Larry playing with his toys.

Another time, Al declared she had found the garden-destroying mole that Grandma had been looking for for years, so she alerted Grandma, who had come storming out of the house with a spade, only to trip and break her wrist. The mole went free once again, and the best bit was when Mum said it wasn't the first time. I could imagine a scoreboard with Mole - fifteen and Grandma - zero etched against it. That was the same week that Mum encouraged me to take my new metal detector to the garden in the hope of it distracting me for an hour. Instead, I ended up unintentionally trying to dig up Grandma and Grandy's deceased dog. Grandma said Grandy would have been laughing at her if he was here because he was in favour of a little gravestone to mark where she was, whereas she had advocated for the natural approach, which nearly saw the return of Bonnie sixteen years after her death.

Back in the present day, I rapped on the door.

'Hello love,' she said as she gave me a proper cuddle, none of that polite pat-pat nonsense. The kind where your lungs creak but you don't care.

'Come on in,' she said turning around. As I crossed the threshold, Sadness, Anxiety, Loneliness and Fear were left at the entrance. I felt my mind start to clear and make room for something else for once. I followed Grandma through to her living room and let myself sink into my usual spot on her sofa. I noticed she already had a cup of tea in my favourite mug of hers, the one with Mickey Mouse on it and shortbread biscuits to go with it. For some reason, a fictional mouse and a biscuit set me off again, and Grandma waited for me to take a second.

'Tell me all about it, love,' she said gently. And just like that, Grandma became my emotional Uber driver, with snacks.

I spent the next few hours telling Grandma everything. R, S and Nina. Even Janice made it into the story, I didn't really have an importance filter, it all just came out. But Grandma listened to every word, no matter the perceived relevance. She listened and watched as my anger ebbed and flowed as I navigated the map of my thoughts, which was so jumbled and disjointed at that point it would have resembled the London Underground wonderfully.

'Now Meg, those words those boys used, they are horrible. But what I'm most worried about is I see you have confidence in what they say,' she said plainly. I thought about it for a moment. 'Those words are subjective. You can gain a great deal from opinion, but one thing it is not is fact, and truly learning and living with that comes with age,' she said as she sipped her tea casually.

'I don't seem to understand anything, though, Grandma,' I said worriedly.

'You're only fourteen, God. When I was fourteen, I was also depressed and didn't have a clue what to do with my feelings either,' she laughed. Thanks, Grandma. We both laughed for a moment, and I wondered what she was thinking, but when the moment passed, I felt my smile fade as my happiness passed the baton back to sadness.

'I don't get why I'm so upset about it all though. I've seen others called worse than me, and they don't seem to care,' I whispered as my voice wobbled again.

'Another one of life's famous lessons, is to learn that we all react differently to different things,' she watched me think about it for a while.

'Listen to your feelings, don't judge them,' she spoke seriously. 'Otherwise, you've tampered with how you actually feel before you've even felt it,' she wiggled her eyebrows on that knowing my tiny mind had just been well and truly blown. I still love a Grandma-ism, they're the best lessons.

'Look here, it will all come out in the wash, love, it always does,' she smiled, to which I smiled wider back.

I only truly learnt the importance of what she had said in my later years. However, what I did manage to take in that moment was a gift unlike any other, hope. She reminded me that better days were coming and looking forward to them got me through the rest of my high school life really. Nothing is ever perfect or plain sailing; however, I know now that hope is a really powerful thing and can change everything. Thanks, Grandma. For everything.

CHAPTER

Seven

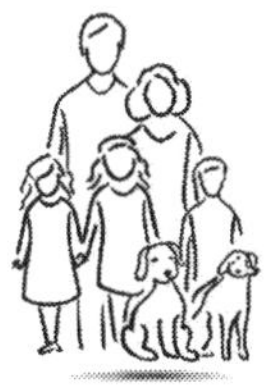

THE YEAR OF MCFLURRIES, BOMB THREATS & TEENAGE HORMONES

Fuelled by Grandma, shortbread, and a sliver of hope, I limped through the rest of the year - emotionally wounded but still somehow in one piece. I was so grateful when it reached its end. GCSE years crept up on me and went a little like this...

September 2015, a month of firsts. It was the first time I went shopping without Mum, and I bought and ate four McFlurries simply because I could. It was the first time I realised being older wasn't all it cracked up to be when I nearly vommed up pieces of mushy Malteaser. I realised being fourteen meant that I felt every emotion but ten times more intense than they used to feel... every emotion, just cranked to level ten, like someone had spilled Red Bull on my puberty dial. It was the first time I developed feelings for another human, which made my day-to-day life much more interesting. Oh, and Mum finally let me join Facebook. Tommy and I reconnected by sending each other a 'wave' every other day. Romance.

October, Shocktober. At the start of the year, Adam was just another boy in my year, a tall and broad build with a fiercely chiseled face. Fast forward a few weeks later, I fancied him so much I would hold my breath whenever he spoke to me, uncontrollably set my cheeks alight when he looked at me and sat next to me in geography that once, pfft, I almost passed out. I used to wear some cheap mascara, the kind that either made you look stunning or made your eyelashes jump ship mid-lesson. I would slap it on on days I was guaranteed to see him and was subsequently gutted when he was off sick. My heart would sink, and I'd be in a mood with no eyelashes left and having to listen to Mr Signa talk about object relativity instead.

Side note: Crushing on Adam shone a light on a much milder version I felt when my stomach flipped three years before in year seven when Tommy looked at me right before he jumped out of the window*.

November blast. The headline 'Explosives found in local high school' spread like wildfire across the county, whereby a girl in year seven brought in a 'replica' grenade for Living History Week. She said she got it from her grandad's attic, but the next thing we knew, the school was on lockdown, and the bomb squad revealed it was very much 'live'. I was getting updates from Al, who'd only joined the school in

September, and the school was almost blown to smithereens. I called Dad to ask if he could pick us up as the school was under bomb threat and there is danger to life, and he told me not to 'wind him up'. Classic. Thanks for that, Dad. On the positive, the bomb squad evacuated the upper part of the school to sort it out. In the end, the worst thing that happened was spending three hours stuck in Mr Hughes' biology class staring at a dolphin brain in a jar on the shelf whilst people were hysterical around me.

December. People were still mean, called me names and made me feel excluded; I may as well have changed my name to Rudolph, given the festive period. Although, much more interestingly, I found out S started hanging around with a new crowd and took up smoking, which surprised me and clearly didn't impress R as he seemed to distance himself, too. It was unheard of; they'd been inseparable since the age of six, although I was part of that too, and we all know how that went.

January. I turned fifteen, and when we returned to school from the Christmas break, the boys seemed to have grown up overnight, physically at least. S had to be about six foot tall, R got broader, and it became apparent that Tommy was one of the first in the year to grow a proper mustache. He shared it on Facebook, and it was a proud moment for all who knew him.

February. S quit smoking!

March. Next-door neighbour Jen knocked on our door at nine o'clock on a random weekday evening to ask Mum if she or any of us had seen Sam's hearing aid? Naturally, Mum said no, considering we hadn't had Sam in the house nor been over theirs in about seven years. Most of his swear words made their way through the walls, in all fairness, but nothing more than that. Hearing aid or no hearing aid, Jen and Sam were still at war and called each other all sorts, but Joe seemed to have fewer and fewer questions for definitions as time went by.

April. S got back on the smoke.

May. I sat on one of my first exams, and I was so nervous that I wrote my surname in the name forename box, forgetting about what I had been called for fifteen years entirely.

June. Jen knocked at the door and updated us on the missing hearing aid. It turned out Sam had eaten his own hearing aid as a 'snack'. Therefore, his parents had to order a custom design with a monster on it to deter him from munching on it in the early hours again. Would he try to take a bite of his glasses next time?

July. Tommy seemed to be the first guy in our year to shave or at least broadcast it, and his mustache was no more. Again, another proud moment for all.

August. Adam found himself a girlfriend, and I'd never spent a sunnier month feeling so grey.

September 2016. I started my final year in comprehensive school. I'd already had the year of hormones, heartbreak, and near explosions. what could possibly go wrong?

*If you've just tuned in, remember that context really is everything.

CHAPTER

Eight

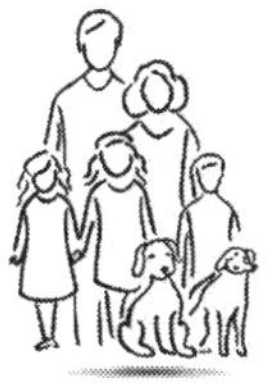

SEGREGATION, SHAKESPEARE AND A SHAMBLES

My last year of GCSEs flew past like a bullet train heading for a distant land. Fast forward to the summer of year eleven, exam season. I'd spent the last two years learning tons of information only to regurgitate it all in a two-hour exam, like one big memory test. Could I remember and apply the memorised knowledge well enough to their questions?

Mid-May, the sun was beating down on an intense day ahead of me, GCSE Biology in the morning and GCSE English Literature in the afternoon. Biology went well; I enjoyed that there was a bigger section on genetics this year. Which left English. I paved the way through a corridor full of anxious students towards the main exam hall. I found us students had different ways of expressing our feelings towards exams. Whichever feeling, though, they all seemed to be exacerbated at the height of exam season.

For example, Drew, who had a hard time managing his anger, seemed to flip out over the most minor things now, including throwing a chair at the breeze, thinking someone was trying to wind him up. Another guy, Adrien, used to get upset over many things, including when we were both practically sobbing over The Titanic in history and had to leave for five minutes to regather ourselves. Now, the poor guy didn't stop crying; he was constantly dehydrated. Mr Butler became known as Butler Buxton due to the supply of Buxton water he supplied Adrien. I was nervous as much as the next person for the pressure of stuffing it up, but simultaneously, exams were simply tickets to better days for me, so the motivation for the reward was greater than the fear of doing them. So, weirdly, I was happy to get stuck in.

Among the many students swarming in the corridors, the head of English, Mrs Townsend-Jones, was guarding the hall doors as if we wanted to enter before our allotted time. She was about four feet tall, but when she opened her mouth, let's just say the sheer volume kept most kids in line, and her height became irrelevant to them, unlike Mr Jase, who was about five feet two inches and quiet - the key word being quiet; he lasted two terms.

'Oi, only year eleven English students can enter; thank you!' She bellowed down the corridor. 'All other students, disappear!' She shooed people away, and she had a lot of huffs as she pissed people off group by group. I meandered through the crowd, but as I went to push the battered-looking door as if by magic, an arm appeared in front of me.

'Only year eleven English students permitted,' she said without any recollection of who I was, even though she had taught me English for the last three years too long.

'It's me, Miss,' I said quickly. 'I'm in this exam,' I went on to say.

'Oi, you, out!' She clicked her fingers and shouted at another boy who entered the door adjacent to the one I was failing to get through. She then turned her angry features back to me.

'I'm literally in your class, Miss!' I couldn't help but giggle a little at this point.

'I think I would know if you were in my class or not, thank you very much, now get on with the rest of your break,' she said in one breath. 'Stay there any longer, and you won't have a break to go to,' she snapped again when I stood still, confused. Forget my break, I wouldn't have A-level college to go to either if she didn't let me in.

I eventually turned around in embarrassment and a little panic for good measure and faced a sea of oncoming students. Then I spotted him instantly. His dark eyes fixed onto mine and he began to laugh as Townsend-Jones continued to bat me away. He gestured for me to come towards him, which felt alien as he'd been avoiding me for the last three years...

'We can go the back way, and you can hide behind me.'

'Thanks R,' I said gratefully. We walked out the way we came in and looped around to the other entrance to the hall. It felt odd to walk beside someone again, especially R. This was my first interaction with him for a long time, and I felt a little warm sensation spread across my chest. He was true to his word and snuck me into the exam hall. Imagine a world where you have to smuggle your mate into an exam. However, it solidified that I was either segregated by my peers or ignored by the teachers. Mrs Townsend-Jones was another thing I wouldn't miss about the place. Truly.

'Good luck, Meg,' R whispered to me as he pulled a few black biro pens and a bottle of water out of his bag.

'Please remove the label; otherwise, it will have to stay in your bag,' an irritated invigilator stated with her eyes narrowed as she inspected the scene in front of her. R wiggled his eyebrows at me over her shoulder as he peeled the label off his water bottle. It seemed it was my turn to laugh from afar, as if Evian was going to give him the answers to why Lady Macbeth killed Duncan. However, my amusement was short-lived as another invigilator snuck up from behind, tapped me on the shoulder and ordered complete silence. My cheeks naturally turned a different shade of embarrassment, to which a big grin stretched R's face out wide as he smirked.

We eventually took our seats and listened to the introduction from the top dog invigilator, who wore a little flat cap. Although he was quite sweet, he explained the exam conditions in a monotonous and rehearsed manner. I zoned out in all honesty, I could only think about was what was going to be on the paper.

'Check your pockets now; if you have any unauthorised possessions, you must hand them in now to avoid disqualification, watches, phones, etc,' he instructed clearly to the room. A soft rustle spread across the hall of all those checking. I padded myself down from head to toe, just in case. I even checked a crease in my shirt in case my phone somehow flew from my bag and landed somewhere. I got some weird looks, but the paranoia was too strong not to. After I confirmed my phone was not in my bra or my pants, I took a few deep breaths before the guy spoke again.

'You have two hours and fifteen minutes,' he glanced at his wristwatch. 'You may turn over your papers and begin.' He turned to write the numbers on the whiteboard, and I realised something crucial: I needed a wee.

Like all the rest, that exam was too important to me, so I managed to suppress the need to empty my bladder for a long while and ploughed through the paper. The next time I looked up, I realised I only had twenty-five minutes left. Twenty-five minutes to write a few sides for the last question felt tight, but what was tighter was my full and extended bladder. The pain began to shoot, no matter how much I readjusted my stance. My focus had shifted from 'how Shakespeare portrays Lady Macbeth as a dangerous character' to thinking how dangerous this could be for me if I were to wee all over the seat, mid-exam, in front of my whole school year. I would die of eternal embarrassment, I was supposed to be sixteen, not six, but nevertheless, the trepidation totally consumed me. I involuntarily shot up my arm, something I'd never done in an exam before. An invigilator arrived almost immediately, like a pop-up advert when you're just trying to play Farm Heroes. They never missed a trick.

'Please, could I go to the toilet, please?' I asked worriedly.

'Can you hold it?' She asked plainly.

'I don't think so,' I replied honestly and fidgeted.

'Follow me,' she instructed. I shot up and followed her gingerly out of the exam hall.

A lot of people seemed to have finished, so naturally, they were watching as a form of entertainment. Maybe I'd fall? Start to cry? Or, most likely, wet myself, my God. I passed one guy, Zac, who looked like he was catching up on sleep; he had his arms folded and his head resting on them. This made me relax a little, and to my detriment, I felt a bit of wee escape and wet my pants a little. I froze on the spot, eyes wide open. A) my sensory side couldn't deal with my clothes being wet in any respect. B) the panic set in. All of a sudden, my worst nightmare was playing out when I looked down to find I was fully wetting myself in front of everyone, and my tights were changing colour. I clicked into flight mode moments too late. One second, I was a GCSE student; the next, a human sprinkler system sprinting out of an exam hall. Thankfully, the toilets were directly opposite the hall, so the invigilator knew I wasn't going elsewhere. I slammed the toilet door shut, but the invigilator threw in a plot twist to an already messy storyline.

'Do not shut that door yet! I need to check you have no notes,' she barked.

'I've-literally-weed-my-self', I spluttered as I opened the door. She looked shifty once she realised I wasn't lying and I had, in fact, soaked my clothes with my own urine. Thanks a bunch, Sandy.

'I will get a teacher to fetch you some lost property clothes,' she said awkwardly. 'But before that, I do need to check that you have no notes,' she said sternly. Notes? Really? If I had a cheat sheet, it would be a soggy mess clinging to my thigh by now. I started to cry and low-key hyperventilated at the thought of ever leaving the toilet cubicle again as I showed her my empty pockets. She even made me take off my jumper to show her nothing was in my shirt. Maybe someone had hidden their phone in their bra, after all.

When I'd stopped having a panic attack, it was twenty-five minutes too late for Shakespeare, so I never answered that last question. Instead, I wet myself, had my first body search and sat in Mrs Griffith's office until half past four so I wouldn't be fed to the wolves, i.e. the student pack. Life hit a bit of a trough there. But what I didn't know then that I do now is that we were in our final year of school and no one actually cared enough. Most importantly, I passed stupid Shakespeare with a B in the end and although I lost ninety-nine percent of my dignity, at least I gained my oldest friend back. R and I started to spend some Saturdays together again. We went to the cinema or for a walk. It was wonderful. I had forgotten what having a friend was all about. I felt content for the first time since year eight, honestly.

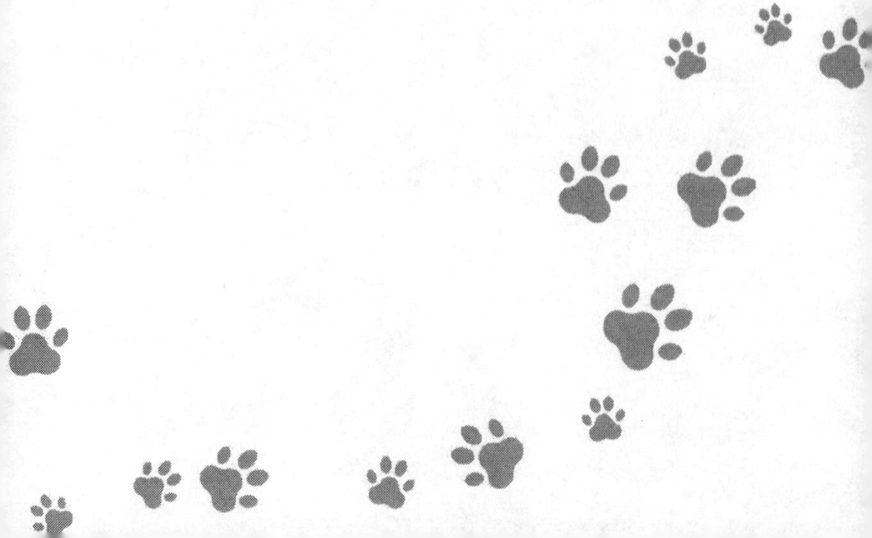

CHAPTER *Nine*

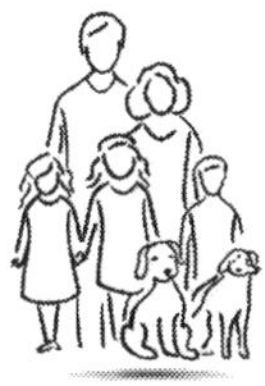

CROESWEN TO COLLEGE

The summer of 2017 was one I'll never forget; sixteen, with no responsibility, and finally free from the prison walls of that bastard high school. Most of my days were spent sunbathing in the garden with the dog or submerged in the bath until the water turned cold and the book pages curled at the edges, but I didn't care, I was free. I was easily pleased and enjoyed no negative feelings for the first time in three long years. The last time I went to Croeswen was when I picked up my GCSE results. I never knew how much I would love seeing the first three letters of the alphabet on pieces of paper. But man, they were amazing and opened the door to a new chapter for me. R and I kept in touch; he sent me a photo of his timetable and a sad-face emoji when I told him I'd applied somewhere else. But he knew. He always knew. By September, I had started at an A-level college, an hour and a half away from Croeswen, which was exactly what I needed. It was a place where no one knew me or had any preconceived judgments of me either. It was a much-needed fresh start, and I felt like Meg again.

CHAPTER
Ten

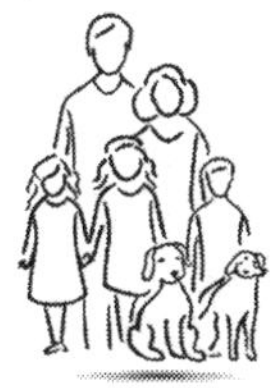

THE A-LEVEL SLAP

September of 2017. I received the almighty A-Level slap across the face, as they called it. I chose Biology, Geography, and Welsh Language, three totally unrelated subjects that reflected the exact degree of coordination (or clearly, lack thereof) I had going for myself. The summer felt like a faraway dream of walking the dog along the beach as the sun disappeared. Now, I didn't even see the sunlight. To be frank, I spent all my days, nights, and actual existence learning, revising, and likely crying. What even is a beach anymore?

October. I was so consumed by my studies that Mum and Dad had to kidnap me from my own revision to have a break. Although I developed Stockholm Syndrome following a twenty-minute walk one evening. Once we got back, I kicked my shoes off and flew up the stairs to be reunited with photosynthesis. I even slept with my revision notes, purely because I'd fallen asleep in the early hours trying to recite a Welsh poem about apartheid (which I didn't even know the English definition of at the time, let alone discuss in another language). Take A-Levels, they said. It would be rewarding, they said. The only thing they'd given me so far was recurring nightmares about mitochondria. Brilliant.

November. My newest friend Daisy called to say she'd passed her driving test and got a Saturday job, all in the same week. She officially became the most highly skilled person I knew.

December. Complete and utter blur.

January of 2018. The mitochondria kept multiplying, and soon enough, the new year hit me - and I turned seventeen. I was pretty shocked I made it this far, and so was the rest of my family. At the grand age of eleven now, Joe congratulated me on staying awake past eleven o'clock on my birthday, and Al said I carried more eye bags than she did after a trip to Asda. Her sarcasm had taken off since she turned fourteen, although that one was brutal honesty at its finest.

CHAPTER
Eleven

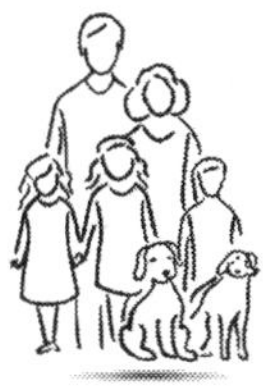

MEGAN OR MAYHEM?

Despite still being happy and grateful that my birthday fell during the Christmas holidays, the educational side of life hit hard again once college resumed in January. A-Levels were just absolute madness most of the time, one day in particular springs to mind. I turned up to Dr C's biology class to find the lab prepped for yet another practical. I didn't enjoy practicals, purely because my seventeen-year-old feet didn't want to stand for longer than five minutes. Everything was exhausting somehow. Anyway, I joined Leon and Sarah and clambered around looking for equipment for an experiment titled:

'Use streak plating to isolate species of bacteria from different cultures.' Thrilling. We all passed the first stage of sterilising our inoculating loops without much difficulty. The only one who ran into trouble was Adam from the back row, who managed to drop his loop onto the Bunsen burner, which toppled over and set his instruction manual on fire. Dr C stormed over, lab coat flying behind her due to the speed. She patted the fire out, coughing and wafting away the smoke. She looked like Julie Andrews in a hazmat nightmare. Best bit? She muttered she'd be lucky if she wasn't just a lab coat by the end of the day, then sent Adam to open all the windows. Adam, who looked like he'd just lost his dog, darted to each window and sat back down, completely silent. I couldn't blame him, he'd ignited a fume in Dr C, and that was for sure. Despite that minor incident, we successfully congregated nine Petri dishes from different cultures. Dr C had us label them before putting them in the incubator, and I remember Leon asking me if it was appropriate to write:

'Leon - Gonorrhoea' or 'Meg - Herpes' on our result dishes. Charming. I reassured him that Dr C likely wasn't growing gonorrhea for her A-Level class, and besides, herpes is a virus, so we wouldn't have to worry about that one. The problem was, Dr C was hovering silently behind us when I said: 'Herpes wouldn't be a problem for me.' She was stealthy, barely four-foot-something and silent on her feet. I didn't stand a chance. Naturally, she reminded us sternly about the assignment brief and told me she had plenty of sexual health resources if I ever needed them. I'd never been so embarrassed in my scholarly life.

'You watch, she'll be screening you for secondary-stage syphilis, given the shade of red your face is, Meg!' Sarah howled. Cheers, mate. To top it off, once we'd cleared the lab, Dr C brought out some example cultures to explain the next steps. There was salmonella, which looked like innocent white bubbles, and staphylococcus, which came in weird yellow shades. Looking would have been far too easy, of course. Leon lost his grip on the salmonella Petri dish, dropped it, and the lid rolled off and some of its contents landed on me. Excellent. Dr C was so livid I was surprised she didn't shoot through the ceiling and teach the rest of the lesson from the roof of the science block. She gave Leon a bollocking and me a thorough cleanse, a referral to the school nurse, and a leaflet to take home to Mum. Brilliant.

> *Hi Mum, here's a letter from Dr C. It explains how I probably won't eat for six days until I know the salmonella is definitely dead, and I've also been referred to the sexual health clinic for syphilis and herpes - even though I promise you, the only thing that's seen me naked since my nappy days is my mirror...*

Once I was finally let go, I spent break watching Sarah eat crisps like it was nothing. It was like having a cold and realising how amazing it is to taste things. You don't miss it until it's gone. After my starved break, I sat through two hours of confusion in Welsh. Our tutor, Aderyn, had decided to use zero English now that we'd hit the five-month mark. I couldn't focus, my mind was still stuck on 'clefydau ac heintiau bacteriol.' Welsh for 'bacterial infections and diseases.' Great.

By the end of the college day, my eyelids felt like they were being held up with matchsticks. I was half-asleep against the science lab wall when I heard: 'Megan or Mayhem?' Did someone just call me Mayhem? 'What are you still doing here?' It was Dr C. God help me. Her thick, short blonde hair had a dent in the front where her goggles usually sat. She wore her long black coat now instead of her white lab coat - which was weird, considering she was all about dissections, explosions, and most recently, fires, STIs, and epidemics...

'I'm just waiting for Daisy, miss,' I said tiredly.

'Right. Well, you get home and relax after today,' she said gently. 'You have a habit of attracting chaos for someone who doesn't look for it.' She smiled like she genuinely felt sorry for me, then walked off, leaving me with a lot of questions, and not many answers.

CHAPTER

Twelve

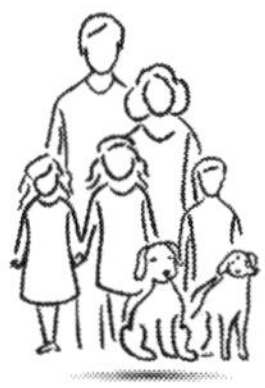

CLASS 'A'-LEVEL TEACHERS

I was just getting accustomed to balancing A-Levels like spinning plates, but the plates were made of ice which of course were melting the whole time...when one random day in March, we were blindsided by Geography George. He formally asked us to start considering options for university.

'But sir, I literally have no idea what I'm doing next week yet,' said a guy named Layton, making a valid point that most of us related to.

'Guys, look, we mention it now, so you have time to think, *before* you start year thirteen in September.' George wore regret in his eyes as he faced a class of panicked teenagers. 'We just want you to attend an open day or two this year so you can see if you can see yourself attending the uni, and, of course, the course of your choice.' He tried to calm a riled class of seventeen-year-olds. He was unsuccessful. The room descended into carnage.

Trinity started crying, Daniel threw his pen on the floor (which Alex picked up and lobbed back at him), and Laila launched into a full-on speech about how doing four A-Levels left her with zero time to visit anywhere. Also, valid. I turned to Dylan, my companion in both form and geography, and smiled worriedly.

'Fuck,' he said, shaking his head. Dylan reminded me of Al, he had that same calming effect on my busy brain, using minimal words. He'd become a good friend early on in college, since we saw each other for about six hours a week in class. He was around five-foot-ten, had a mop of bright blonde hair, and used to wear knitted jumpers, which killed me. How a seventeen-year-old lad managed to pull off grandad chic was beyond me. I started laughing at the pure dismay on his face as George began explaining the world of UCAS, but by the end of it, neither of us could stop.

Later that day, Dylan took me to McDonald's during our break. He'd passed his driving test early and was an actual natural behind the wheel.

'So, what are you thinking?' I asked, slumping back in the passenger seat.

'Well, I want to be a lawyer eventually. It's good money, good life,' he said confidently.

'But then...I feel it's a lot of pressure and work. I don't know if I could hack my whole life into work.' He pondered as he hit the accelerator on the dual carriageway.

'I'm with you. I've never seen myself doing anything other than something healthcare related. Being a paramedic has always been the idea, but then... is the pay worth the stress?' Dylan screwed up his face with uncertainty.

'Exactly.' I answered my own question. 'Probably not.'

'Maybe be a teacher, Meg?' he offered, deadpan.

'Pfff, no. Imagine me trying to keep our classes in line,' I scoffed.

'Maybe I'll teach geography. I'm alright at it,' he shrugged. 'But I'd never be as committed as George.' He laughed. 'Imagine that...' We both cracked up at the thought. See, George cycled to work every day. From Bridgend. Yes, cycled, three hours each way. I couldn't even cycle to Grandma's house five minutes down the road without getting a wedgie and walking like I'd been impaled, let alone ride six hours a day. Mental. But that was George, in the best way possible. He looked shattered most days, hung his hi-vis vest on top of the totem pole he brought back from Canada, and was just a damn good human. He genuinely cared for each of us and had this effortless gift for all things geography.

I'll forever be thankful to George, Aderyn, and even Dr C (eventually) for showing me that not all teachers don't give a shit. Aderyn used to set up FaceTime sessions so we could practice conversational Welsh, even picked up once while getting her nails done. We all sat there talking about sexual health in Welsh. Thankfully, the salon was fully English speaking. So, we were told. And then there was Dr C, Mary Poppins of the science department. Everything practically perfect. But again, it was because she cared. I remember crying my eyeballs out once after a particularly complex lesson on gaseous exchange, panicking over how the hell everyone else seemed to understand. She made me a hot chocolate, broke the topic down, reminded me it was essentially just the science of breathing, and I left feeling like I could maybe survive A-Level Biology after all. I'd never had teachers like them. And I haven't since.

CHAPTER *Thirteen*

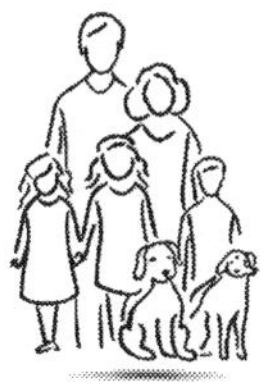

THE DAY A GIANT VAGINA HIJACKED MY CAREER PLANS

Seventeen and a half years on the planet, with naivety as my best friend, I'd had my heart set on being a paramedic since I was about six. Apparently, this ambition bloomed when I resuscitated my Tweenies after orchestrating a seven-car pile-up at the foot of my bed using vehicles stolen from my brother's room. Or maybe it started when I cut holes into my Cabbage Patch's mesh-like stomach with Mum's nail scissors, just so I could sew them back up again. Looking back now, I do wonder if these were early psychopathic tendencies, but thankfully, I was far more interested in fixing people. Just to clarify. Anyway, armed with childhood dreams and absolutely no clue about the real world, I arrived at Sheffield University for an open day in Paramedic Science.

I peeled off my coat and tried to fold myself into the seat groove of the lecture hall, where countless arses had clearly done the same. I scanned the tall, empty ceiling and stark white walls, broken only by the odd scattered poster. One in particular caught my eye, a mental health awareness one, corners curled and hanging on by a thread of blue tack. I didn't know it yet, but that limp poster would become a visual representation of my emotional state on multiple occasions to come. Blissfully unaware, I glanced at Al. She met my smirk with her own. Classic silent humour. But the moment was broken when a tall man in a green uniform took the stage.

'I'm Rich. Paramedic and lead lecturer for Paramedic Science here at the university,' he boomed into the mic. I looked over at Al, whose face had morphed into a sarcastic 'no shit' expression. I ducked my head to hide my laugh as Mum shot me a sharp look that said: don't you dare. I'd already lost track of who the other lecturers were and instantly fell behind. But I was quickly snapped back by Rich's barrage of stats about the job: paper cuts reported as severed fingers, calls for actual cardiac arrests and strokes flooding the system all at once. I looked around. Everyone wore the same expression, concentrated fear. That's when the sinking feeling started. I don't know what I expected, but the stress sat in my gut like a stone. Maybe it was just youthful naivety. Maybe it was something deeper.

Rich carried on about the course itinerary, job prospects, and what we'd need to get in. By the end of it, my eyes were glassy, not with inspiration, but with sympathy for the version of myself that wanted this. He spoke about elderly patients waiting for beds in awful conditions, and how often that was the reality.

'Any questions, folks? Big or small, fire away!' He grinned, proud of himself. Pretending he hadn't just traumatised a room of mostly teenagers. No one moved. No one spoke. Which only made the internal panic louder. I came close to asking Rich if you could adopt an elderly person, like how you adopt an orangutan from the rainforest. Would they send you a cuddly toy gran? No, Meg. No, they wouldn't. You'd probably get arrested for abduction. That's when I realised I'd entered an advanced stage of stress: random, absurd mental distractions. The place where orangutans and elderly people merge into one single unhinged coping strategy.

By the time I came back to earth, people were putting on their coats. Leaving? Already? Shit, I'd basically missed the whole thing. I turned to find Al and my parents packing up, and just like that, I was out of there faster than I'd run for the Chinese before closing the week before. I wore the slap of reality red raw across my cheeks. And everyone knew it.

'Well, that wasn't what I was expecting,' Mum said gently. 'There's got to be more rewarding moments than not, Meg. Remember that.'

'Nope. I can't do this,'I said, flustered. I turned to Al.

'Not for you, Meg.' Her words hit me blankly.

Then came the final phase of panic: fixing it. Dad, ever the emotionally fluent tribal leader, jumped into action.

'Let's check out other degree options while we're here,' he offered, already marching ahead. We ended up touring half the bloody campus. Each course was judged, ruthlessly:

- English - Pass. I told Shakespeare where to shove it back in the day.
- Art - If paper-mâché willies flung across the room count as art, then maybe.
- History - Last thing I remember was crying during Titanic in year nine and not getting on a boat for three years.
- Maths - Swam away from that in year seven.
- Biology - Loved it at A-Level thanks to Dr C. But the recurring mitochondria nightmares? No thanks.

We skipped through until we hit a door on the second floor decorated with mountains, volcanoes, all things geography. The clouds parted. A holy glow emerged. My family trailed behind, already aware of my obsession with physical geography. I stepped inside. Breathed in tectonic plates, exhaled population density charts. Bliss. Then Dad lobbed a grenade.

'Where's it going to take you, though, Meg? You'll be in piles of debt to work in a shop in Japan or something,' he paused, 'Paramedic Science guarantees you a job.' Ouch.

'Geography. Filth,' Al added, now no longer soothing my nerves, just tap dancing on them.

'People can do other things than be in the NHS, mind,' I snapped. Mum, ever the negotiator, tried a new tactic.

'Midwifery's over there, Meg. What about that? You'd make a lovely midwife!' The room was empty, so I figured, why not? I tiptoed in.

That's when I saw it. Front and centre on a table the size of a small country: a giant plastic vagina. Every department had an emblem. Geography had a globe. Biology had a skeleton. Midwifery had...this. I whipped around and silently mouthed to my family: 'We. Are. Leaving.' Before Al could reply, a voice boomed behind me.

'Welcome! Don't be shy, come on in!' Goddamn it. Before I could bolt, Mum sauntered in like she'd just spotted a handbag on sale, grabbed me by the arm, and spun me back toward the black hole. And I don't mean metaphorically. I mean... if you just opened this book on this page and saw the words 'giant black hole,' you might assume we were discussing space. Nope. We're talking anatomical display pieces. Turns out, black holes exist closer than you think and reside in most of the population. Annie, the friendly midwife, emerged in blue scrubs, tottering towards us with a smile. She launched into a passionate talk about becoming a midwife, all while the giant plastic vagina sat proudly between us like it had earned a degree itself. Eventually, she asked the dreaded question:

'How long have you wanted to pursue this lifestyle?' *Lifestyle?* What is this, a yoga retreat?

'Six years,' I blurted, face on fire. We all know it had been six seconds. Annie lit up with joy. The guilt rose. By some miracle, another student walked in, fresh meat, and I seized the opportunity to escape. I grabbed a leaflet, nodded like I was deeply inspired, and left. As I passed the door, I heard Annie offering the poor girl a chance to do a vaginal exam. Nope. We were done.

We piled into the car. I shoved my headphones in and sank into self-doubt. Geography was easy, my natural skill. Paramedic science was the dream, but that voice in my head kept saying it wasn't for me. I looked down at the midwifery flyer and, for the first time, let my mind wander freely. No judgment. No plan. Just... open thought. It was hard letting go of an idea I'd built my whole identity around. But change doesn't wait for your permission, it just happens. I realised growth only comes when you get comfortable with the uncomfortable. And as I envisioned myself empowering women through one of the most emotional and meaningful moments of their lives... maybe, just maybe, I'd give it a go.

CHAPTER
Fourteen

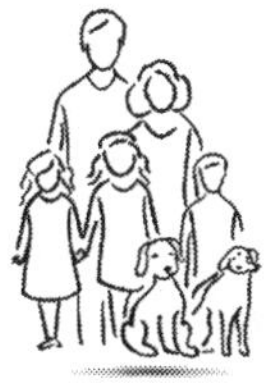

DRIVEN TO THE BRINK (AND SOMETIMES THE PAVEMENT)

Although I was stuck at a crossroads for my career, my A-levels wouldn't pass themselves. Life got more intense, and, in a few months, I had learnt how to recite anaerobic and aerobic respiration in the shower, backwards. I learnt how to walk on a beach, analyse coastal defences and name case studies around the globe. I learnt how to have a conversation in Welsh with no English so much so, I started to think in Welsh from time to time. My favourite example of this is when someone pissed me off so much that I muttered 'pen-coc' under my breath, the wondrous Welsh word for dickhead. I learnt that I could do difficult things and passed my first year of A-levels with flying colours, fatigue and a little dread for year thirteen for good measure.

Onwards and upwards, I used my time off to learn how to drive. I kept comparing it to Mario Kart (but with insurance this time) to stop myself freaking out behind the wheel. The only differences were that you generally avoided throwing things at people, smashing into other people's cars and going off-road. Although we all know plenty of us who have done at least one of those things if not all three. Anyway, my instructor was an older man from the valleys who came with great reviews. However, he fell asleep in the passenger seat once, and I was so terrified that I just kept driving in second gear until he woke up and wondered why we were halfway to Hereford, and the smell of burning was in the air. Mum and Dad weren't best pleased, to say the least, and instead, I started going out with Dad when college restarted. Dad had a great way of staying calm and clearly instructing me in a way that didn't overwhelm me. We did a drive or two a week in between college. A couple of journeys in, I drove his car to try out an automatic, which was kind of like buying a ready meal and heating it up in the microwave; the hard bit was done for you. I loved it an realised an automatic would definitely be the car for me someday (when I'd won the lottery it seemed). We cruised down the dual carriageway and meandered around the suburbs back to base.

'To the right a bit, Meg,' he said casually as we were one or two streets away from home.

'Okay?' I turned the wheel slightly to the right, and with that, a thump of the wheels coming off the curb and back on the road emerged.

'Lovely,' he said, and we both felt the world looked level again rather than from a slanted perspective. I was cruising half on the curb.

Despite my newfound skills after Dad started coaching me, it took a few attempts to pass the practical test but hear me out. Here it goes; the first time, I had a panic attack and had to turn around and book it for another day; the second time, I simply couldn't parallel park without assaulting the curb, the third time I went too fast around a corner and the examiner had to hold onto the door (fair enough), the fourth time I went blank on a hill start and rolled down rather than up, and finally the fifth I smashed it with perfect marks. Silver linings, I guess.

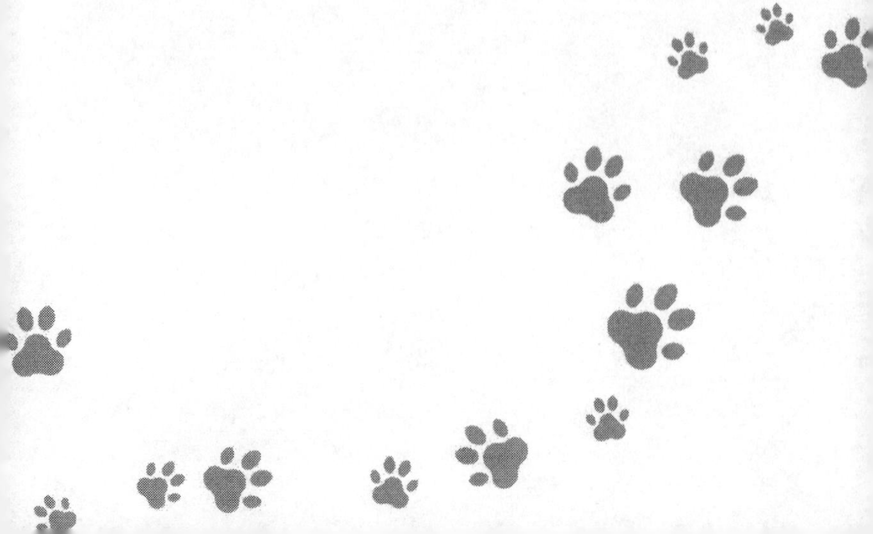

CHAPTER *Fifteen*

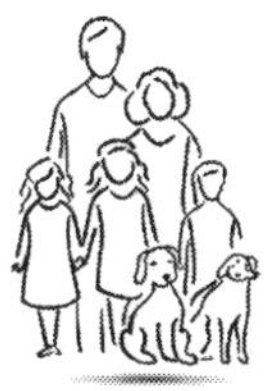

CAREER PATH: DECIDED BY A COIN, QUESTIONED FOR LIFE

I was still shocked when we received the breakdown of our results and individual exam marks; I got full marks for geography and George called me his little prodigy. Dr C scheduled a meeting for us all to discuss our results, no matter the outcome, and discuss goals for the impending year. Whereas Aderyn told us that she would be toasting a glass of wine to us all that evening. I felt the warmest feeling knowing my teachers were behind me; I had family and friends beside me and a hopeful future ahead of me. It was a tremendous alleviation.

Following a short time for celebration and recuperation from the year preceding it, September quickly came around and marked my final year of my school days. The weeks steamrolled by, and the need to apply to universities came inevitably closer. This also meant I had an important decision to make. Paramedic Science was cut off since that open day with Rich, so I forgot about it completely. I thanked my gut for that one. My heart held onto geography, but I also had a new love interest, midwifery. My brain, however, wasn't so decisive. I spent weeks ruminating on their advantages and disadvantages and where they could take me. At the age of seventeen, ultimately deciding what I'd like to do for the majority of my life was highly intense and a little nonsensical. Nevertheless, I was continuously preoccupied with weighing up my options. I walked the dog up to the top of the Brecon Beacons and thought, yes, geography it is. Breathtaking views, the composition of the landscape and how it came to be. However, I saw a pregnant person on the way back down and imagined the craziness of helping her birth her child. Like her brand-new human. Madness. I felt like I needed a career with flagrant aspects in it to feed my brain's need for constant stimulation. Which way to go?

'Mum! I dunno what to do anymore,' I huffed as I held myself in a ball in the corner of the sofa. Mum looked up from counting out some change for Joe to take to school for a mufti day.

'Look, Meg,' She also huffed. 'You've always wanted to care for people; that's always been a common theme. I know which I'd pick for you, but it's not about me.' With that, she hurried after Joe. I stared at the table for so long my eyes glazed over. I blinked a few times to regain focus and spied a fifty-pence piece that Mum had left behind. The next thing

I knew, I'd gotten out of my self-pity ball, grabbed the coin and chucked it in the air, putting the fate of my life onto that fifty-pence piece. Heads for geography and tails for midwifery. UCAS applications were only three weeks away, and I remained indecisive. So there, cupped in my hands, was that fifty-pence piece that held the decision of a lifetime. The responsibility of even finding out was bad enough, so I put it under my bed and left it there for when I had psyched myself up enough to find out.

When I finally came around to it, I slowly peered under my bed to reveal my twist of fate. Despite the initial shock, I felt somewhat relieved to have a decision made. By the twenty-second of October, I'd applied to five different universities for midwifery. What had I done? I'd only picked up a leaflet and fifty p?

CHAPTER *Sixteen*

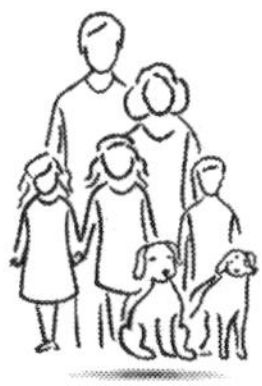

MISSION: IMPROBABLE

A few weeks after I based my life choices on a coin, two universities invited me for an interview, two of them never got back to me at all, and one rejected me flat out. Charming. Firstly, Bangor University's interview. It was an indisputable disaster. Start to finish, a shambles. The train journey took longer than the average time I spent sleeping every night, and the ticket cost approximately eighty percent of my savings at the time. If that wasn't enough, the taxi never showed up the morning of the interview, so Mum and I had to leg it through the middle of North Wales without any knowledge of the area at all. The interviewers asked for my passport, to which I joked about saying that I'd only popped up from South Wales. They didn't share the humour; instead, I got a telling-off for not checking my emails for the requirements on the interview day. No matter how much I tried to explain that I had not received the email (which I truly hadn't), they called me 'irresponsible and were disappointed I didn't tell the truth'. Naturally, I foresaw the letter of rejection before they even sent it. Mum and I laughed it off for every one of the nine-hours that the train took to get us home. She was also pleased that I hadn't chosen geography (or rather, the coin hadn't chosen geography), given my lack of capability to map read. Call it fate, but I received an email on the train home from Worcester Uni inviting me for an interview. Mum and I roared with laughter at the pure irony.

'It will be easy!' Mum's face was bright red. 'Just do not do anything you did this time!' She laughed wholeheartedly as I face-planted the table in front of me and relived the carnage of the day. Thanks, Mum; that was precisely what I needed to do.

CHAPTER Seventeen

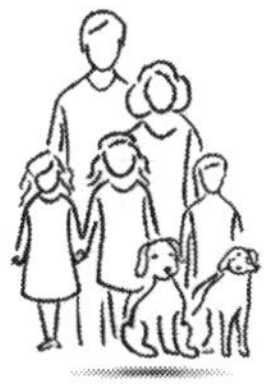

CONDITIONAL OFFER, UNCONDITIONAL CHAOS

Year thirteen was intense in its most basic form. Aside from trying to survive my A-levels, I had universities to navigate. Thankfully, I achieved the opposite of Bangor's interview at Worcester and received my singular offer from them to study 'BSc Hons Midwifery' in September 2019. Imagine five unis, one offer. But I guess it only took one to say yes. Despite the relief of my only yes, the pressure was on when the conditional offer included smashing my A-levels with three B grades. Shit.

The last year remains the quickest year I have perceived to date. I spent my days either at college or with my head so far in textbooks, and I'm surprised I didn't become one. I didn't see any of my friends for months as they were almost guaranteed to be doing the same. The students weren't the only ones feeling the rising pressure; the teachers felt it too. Dr C was more uptight as the exam season came around, but that's probably because she spent all her time coaching us. I had a few hot chocolate and cry sessions with her during the build-up, notably after our practical exam, where I went to slice my piece of potato with the blunt knife provided, and its rubbery texture rejected the piece, and it went flying straight past the examiner's head. She had to go and find me a new one from the other class. It was all stress, no starch.

Opposing stress, Aderyn, on the other hand, took a different approach to more relaxed classes; she asked us what we wanted to work on as final brush-ups before it all came to an intense peak. This involved a discussion about the latest plot twist in Emmerdale but in total Welsh. Get eighteen-year-olds gossiping about soaps, genius.

Meanwhile, George's eyes became more bloodshot as he held revision classes until six most nights. One Friday night, when I asked him about my case study potentially being wrong and that I might have messed up over two thousand rock measurements, I remember how he rubbed his forehead and said, 'I think this is a future George and Meg problem to deal with, go and have a good weekend and we will sort it all on Monday' a quote I rely on to this day; 'it's a future Meg problem.' Those were the days of finding the silver linings in the academic tornado. My nights weren't much better; they were spent mostly on the exam board's website, attempting past papers for practice. One of the most prominent memories to look back on was when I bashed out a biology past paper at two am, and one of the answers I gave was 'ammonia'. However, at the bottom of all eleven other possible answers, the WJEC had legit written 'NOT AMMONIA' in capital letters. Bastards. I literally slammed my laptop shut and used it as a pillow instead. Mum asked what on earth I was doing when she found me in the morning, seized from sleeping in my chair, head on my buzzing laptop. I cried and told her it was all ammonia's fault. I remember she patted me on the back and dragged me away for the day, but we never mentioned ammonia again.

Despite flying potatoes, thousands of rock circumferences and ammonia, to my absolute stupefaction and utmost relief, all the hard work paid off. I achieved ABB. Geography was the A, and I had a moment of regret for not sticking with what I knew best for my next move in life. It was on results day that I truly realised my life was about to be turned on its head, and I was going to enter a totally unknown world. And despite the many tears I had spent crying an A-level river, I was going to miss Dr C, George, and Aderyn. I owe them all a lot, to say the least.

PART 2

University (essentially more growing up)

YEAR 1

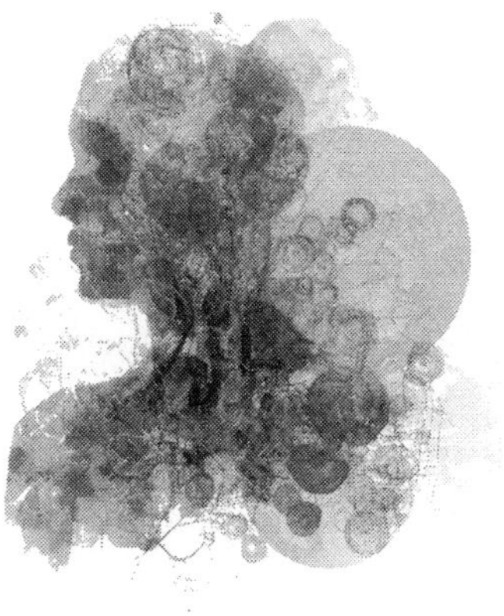

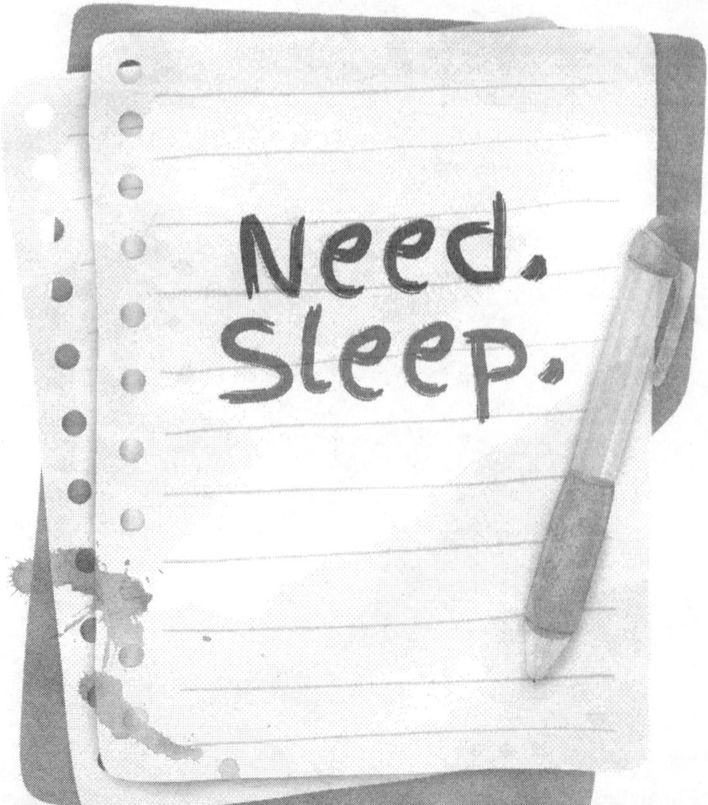
Need.
Sleep.

CHAPTER Eighteen

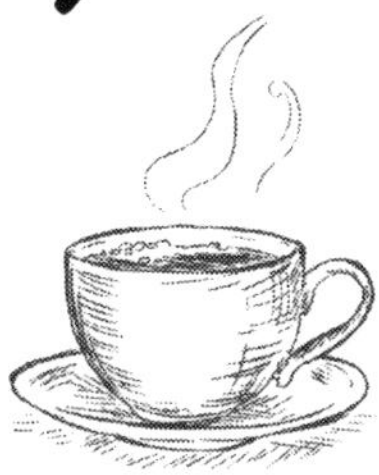

NO ONE WARNED ME ABOUT THE TOAST

'Morning Meg! Big day!' Mum said spritely. I gave a wry smile in return. Thirty-first of August meant I had to reluctantly move to university. I wasn't feeling it. I initially felt pride as I had achieved what I had always strived for. Still, the closer September loomed, a diminutive feeling of dread slowly swelled inside my stomach.

'You'll be alright, Meg,' Dad said as he got up from one of the chairs in the kitchen. 'You'll always have this place,' he said as he stuck his head in the washing machine, looking for his polo shirt.

'Try and eat, Meg,' Mum said, sliding a bowl of cornflakes in front of me. I sat at the breakfast bar, stirring them like I was conducting a very depressing symphony. Even my favourite sustenance had turned traitor. From the laminate floor came the familiar tap-tap-tap of paws on patrol. Marshall was making his rounds. We'd rescued him after losing M&M, once we were ready to risk dog hair and heartbreak again. What we got was a dalmatian - the polar opposite of a sheepdog. We'd gone from disciplined and hardworking to... a polka-dotted liability. He trotted through the house like a spotted security guard, checking every room before zeroing in on me - or, more accurately, on my cornflakes.

'What do you want my darling?' I asked him in a pitch much higher than I would speak to any human. He stuck his chocolatey brown nose up and sniffed vigorously. I rested my head on my hands and felt nothing but sadness. What was wrong with me? I barely felt sadness these days. I rubbed my eyes and gazed up at the ceiling, my sorrow evident. My brain couldn't seem to be able to resist firing questions at me; Why leave a very happy place? Why try and fix something that is not broken? Tears at bay, I looked down at my amalgamated cornflakes and milk, then to the dog who had been drooling, and created a smear of thick saliva on my right sock. Brilliant.

After getting rid of the cornflake pat and changing my socks, we had to go. I chucked a hoodie on and shivered as I migrated gradually to the car. I waved goodbye to Al, Joe, and Marsh, who were all in the window watching as we packed the last of my bags. Dad drove us away, and for once in my life, I didn't feel like talking. I decided to create solitude by burying my AirPods deep within my ears for the journey. I absorbed myself in my own world and watched the countryside flash by as a continuous blur as Dad drove us further and further away from home. Now and then, my mind came out of its isolation and recognised the growing feeling of disquietude devouring my stomach. However, I fought it and told myself to refocus on the melodious voices of One Direction, telling me things would all be fine.

After what felt like an eternity, we arrived at the gates of Worcester University. It was just as endearing as their brochure had depicted it. Only this time, the paths were lined with blue tents that read, 'Accommodation check-in' and aficionados were wearing radiant blue t-shirts and baseball caps that complemented the Worcestershire logo. Anyway, as we turned into the gates, my despondent eyes were drawn to the woodland which surrounded the long, stony trails that lead visitors towards the campus. It was pretty. But I didn't care for how appealing the woodland was. South Wales was more so. I'd have given anything to see Swaying Sue stumble back to her house opposite ours after her trip to the pub or hear Slimy Sam calling his mum a slug and hearing her get her own back.

A long way away from Swaying Sue and Slimy Sam, Dad proceeded to drive us past the shrubbery where hedges garnished with small yellow flowers began to supersede it. Encased within them, there was a relatively small building in the centre, signposted 'Health and Social Science' block. I took a sharp, deep breath as we entered the building. We were greeted by many of the friendly Worcesterian members of staff, and we found ourselves joining a rather lengthy line of fresh students. Was that what I was, a fresher? I wasn't sure whether I wanted to cry or cringe at the thought. Turns out, I went on to do both a few hours later, crying, feeling as though my life was over and cringing at the cliche that I had become.

'Name, please,' a short lady with an even shorter temper fired at me as I got to the front of the queue. I sensed a great deal of irritation from her.

'Megan,' I quickly blurted out, then wondered if it was the right answer.

'Course?' She shot just as rapidly back.

'Midwifery,' I said nervously, as though she was going to tell me I was wrong. She loaded my image onto her screen for the world to see, and I could have died with embarrassment. Over the summer, I received a letter requesting a passport-like photo of me for my ID card. I took it seriously and made it a proper passport photo, expressionless. I could see her pupils were fixed upon my photo, and then they flicked up to my face and back down. I side-eyed the other desks on either side of me and saw the other students didn't take the 'passport' instruction quite as I had. The photo of the boy next to me was like a personal act of publicity for himself.

He was wearing a pair of bright, yellow, triangular-shaped glasses that he had just casually resting on his nose. His eyebrows were stretched to capacity as if they were reaching up for his hairline. His smile was so widespread across his cheeks that they may have had to crop it, so it fitted on the card. My brain couldn't help but give him an internal round of applause. Turning back to my face of thunder, my interior applause immediately ceased. I turned to the other guy's photo on the other side of my station. His picture showed his whole upper torso; he was standing in a solid stance as if looking forward past my shoulders into my past life, with his arms flexed in front of him. He wore a posh Ralph Lauren top and had unquestionably made an ample effort.

'Think you missed the memo, Meg!' Mum chuckled. 'You look fuming,' she said as she dissected my newly printed ID card.

'No, Mum, actually stop,' I said through a nervous smile, the first smile of the day. 'I swore it said passport-type thing,' my voice slowly tailed off as the woman at the desk was now locking her piercing eyes with mine.

'It did say passport, as in passport *size*,' she decided to clarify after clipping my card to a University of Worcester lanyard. There was no getting out of this now. I sadly slung the lanyard over my head and walked out of the student services building with my depression campaign strapped to my chest. Who was the boring one now?

After spending forever trying to unlock the door to my new room, I finally figured out my depressed ID card was also, in fact, my key card. So, this meant I couldn't chuck it to the bottom of my sock drawer for the foreseeable. Excellent. What was more disturbing was finding all of the walls doused in sour green paint.

It gave me migraines with lime green auras just looking at them. Who on earth would consciously choose bile as a decorative option? Anyway, I met the other five girls in 'Oak' halls, and we spent the first week of September getting to know each other. Since I was living with four other strangers around the clock, I felt I knew what they meant on Big Brother now when the contestants said living twenty-four/seven with strangers felt like hyper speed. Although, they also said the same thing to justify a marriage proposal after two weeks. Gladly avoiding marriage proposals and evictions, a few things I had learnt in the first seven days of living together were; Lula's favourite topic was by far, Lula; Harriet spent most of her time on FaceTime; Amy had her girlfriend up to stay, and I hadn't seen her door open since; and as for Jordan, she was barely there. I'd had beans on toast, cheese on toast and, to the rest of the girl's disgust, tuna on toast. Times were hard, and I was desperate, okay? By the time we hit seven days since we moved in, I felt like my body composition was solely bread as I lived the stereotypical student life.

CHAPTER *Nineteen*

BREAKING THE ICE

After two weeks of surviving on toast in its many forms, I finally expanded my diet to include ready meals, basically cardboard with a hint of microwave. Anyway, after time to settle in, if you could call it that, the Monday marking our first day at uni was upon us. We all gathered in the hallway to leave united as the girls from Oak. Strength in numbers and all of that. To mark the occasion, I shoved on a jersey jumper and leggings and knocked my hair back into a low bun. I was the first waiting outside the door, clicking my watch obsessively to ensure we wouldn't be late. A couple of minutes passed, and I finally heard a click of one of the doors.

Lulu emerged from her room looking like Beyonce, to which my jaw dropped a little. She had her long black hair slicked back. Was it hair gel? Witchcraft? I didn't care that hair wasn't moving for anyone. My hair only stayed stationary like that when I was on day five of not washing it. Whatever it was, natural grease or expensive hair gel, she looked stunning fair play to her. Harriet wasn't far behind her; she came out of her room with a face full of makeup and a skin shade darker than yesterday? She failed to mention the fake tan until I mentioned questionable marks on my coat. At least we could all follow the fake tan trail if she got herself lost around campus. Amy joined the congregation in her oversized hoodie and jeans, which made me feel a little better, meanwhile, Jordan wore a short, neon pink top with dark, flared jeans.

'I think you look grand, Jord,' I said as she affirmed that it was her favourite outfit from the nineties.

'That took us exactly three minutes and twenty seconds,' Amy declared, assessing her watch as we walked from Oak Halls to the university campus.

'Now that's my kind of walk,' Jordan said happily, to which we all laughed. We all looked up at the uni, which would be the start of a lengthy and challenging journey over the next few years. The university itself looked fairly modernised, an assemblage of many smaller buildings with swarthy brown brick exteriors. Brightly coloured shrubbery traced the outskirts of the buildings, and a few wooden picnic benches were dotted between them. Aesthetically pleasing, it was an inviting way to start. However, the interior looked like every other sixth-form college. Shiny brown flooring and blue classroom doors which looked like they had seen better days.

'Looks like we need to head this way, girls,' Lulu drew her timetable out from her trendy Zara bag and directed us to the west of the main block. Harriet and Amy walked alongside Lulu whilst Jordan, and I brought up the rear. We made our way through crowds of students, just like us. One boy stood with the map scratching his head whilst another group we saw a few times as they kept switching the direction in which they were walking. Eventually, we found the lecture hall, marking where it would all begin. Lecture hall one: Midwifery Sept 19 cohort, a flat screen flashed above the quadruple doors granting access to it. I felt a congregation of nerves buzz at the pit of my stomach. I flashed my eyes across to the others, and they looked like I felt. Whatever we had let ourselves in for, at least, for now, we would do it together.

'Come in, everyone,' a short woman with profound grey hair welcomed us as she opened one of the four doors. 'How lovely to see so many of you,' she went on to say as she ushered us into the lecture hall and urged us to take a seat. We all shuffled in nervously and took seats in the groups we came in with. The lecture hall made the thirty of us look miniature, and I remember thinking it could have housed our crowd three or four times.

'Everyone seems a lot older you know!' Amy whispered to the rest of us.

'You're right; only a few look our age!' Harriet whispered hard in response as she returned from surveying the ascending rows of people around us. The low hum of chattering stopped once the screen flashed to a PowerPoint presentation titled 'What does midwifery mean to you?'. The first question of the degree, and I didn't have the answer, what had I actually gotten myself in for?

Our lecturers, Lynsey and Annie (who I remember enticed me all that time ago at the open day), introduced themselves and outlined the plan for the year ahead. It comprised many aspects of theoretical and practical midwifery that I hadn't even considered. Some things I hadn't even heard of were VBACs, hypnobirthing and even vaginal seeding. Could you plant a vagina? Imagine a little pot on your windowsill, and the landlord asks what it is, 'Oh yes, just my little vaginal seedling...' Anyway, Lynsey and Annie reassured us we would know all of this someday. They went on and discussed assignments, deadlines and grading systems which seemed to cause an apprehensive stir amongst their audience. Receptive to this, Lynsey swiftly moved the conversation onto practical placements and what to expect. We would all start with six weeks of community placement to lay down the fundamentals of midwifery and move on to hospital-based work after this. After an hour of information overload, we were sent on a twenty-minute break. Three of the five of us enjoyed it; meanwhile, Jordan and I speculated about what was ahead of us (although, honestly, I can tell you now, we had no idea).

We all returned to the lecture hall with a coffee and a cake, and I noticed that almost everyone else had done the same. Evidently, we had all felt the hit of reality this morning. Re-claiming our seats in the hall, I saw that Lynsey was perched on a chair, still pecking at that never-ending bunch of grapes she had started about three hours before. Annie, however, had opened a family-size bag of Skittles. An elite choice.

'Welcome back!' Lynsey exclaimed. 'And well done for coming back,' Annie added. Congratulations on returning after one lecture? What did that say about the actual degree?

'So, we've discussed what midwifery training means to the government, but what does it mean to you? What brought *you* here?' Lynsey asked rhetorically. 'So, midwifery, to me, is all about the physiology of life itself. It's remarkable, terrifying, exhilarating and heartbreaking. All at the same time,' Lynsey had captured everyone's attention, and I felt like I couldn't carry on munching through my lemon muffin.

'We ask you this because although midwifery can be a wondrous profession, it can be awfully hard,' Annie said carefully. 'So, to help move through this, we have found that when students reflect on their initial motivations for wanting to become midwives, we get positive results for retention,' Annie supported Lynsey.

'Please take a moment to jot down your inspiration for starting this journey for yourself on the post-it note we have left on each of your workstations. What helped you decide to sit in front of us today? Why midwifery? And why now?' Lynsey encouraged us to think deeper. That bloody fifty pence loomed at the front of my brain until I forced myself to think a little harder. That image momentarily went to the back of my head, and another rationale came to light. I decided to pursue this degree because I wanted to feel a sense of importance and helping others was always on the agenda. I wrote, 'To be the reason someone felt safe/had a better experience than they could have had.' Folding the Post-it note into a tiny cube, we were all told to keep it somewhere safe. I scribbled 'for a rainy day' on the tiny cube and slotted it into the back pocket of my backpack*.

'Now that you have reflected on why you came, we need to talk about some light realities of the job!' Lynsey said cautiously.

'Some of you married? Boyfriends? Girlfriends?' She asked us all. Almost everyone put their hands up or nodded their heads in agreement. 'Well, this degree is dreadfully time-consuming and will take every inch of your being sometimes.' Immediate internal collapse. We expected a warm welcome, not an academic Hunger Games.

'Marriages often end. Boyfriends/girlfriends will leave you.' Annie supported her collegue. Most of us looked shocked, but for once in my life I was glad I didn't have a significant other to lose.

'The reason why is that you will change. The person who is sitting here now won't be the same person tomorrow, let alone in three years time,' Lynsey delivered with caution.

'Oh, and a lot of you will drop out,' Annie added. 'Being a midwife is not for everyone, and some of you just won't have the stomach for it,' she said sternly. I felt my eyebrows involuntarily creep up my forehead in shock whilst other faces were dripping concern. For the first time, I saw bravery in the people around me and in myself.

'Right, enough serious talk now,' Lynsey clapped her hands together. She smiled casually as if the truths from her discussion were nonchalant. 'An ice breaker for you all,' she clicked the slide and a title read 'Alternative names for vagina'. Silence. Crickets. My brain? Offline.

'As you can see from the slide on the screen,' Lynsey chuckled. 'I thought we'd finish off with a fun exercise as we've had a full-on day today. Lots of information to take in!' She took a sharp breath in. 'So, let's go around the class. Everyone gives me your name and a different name for vagina!' Lynsey looked like she was enjoying this way too much. 'I'll start it off,' she shrugged, 'Fanny!' She publicised. Some of us laughed quietly.

'Vagina,' Annie stated the obvious and Lynsey rolled her eyes affectionately in response.

'You're up next. Please provide your name and synonym!' Lynsey pointed at a girl with her sunglasses perched on top of her head.

'Alina,' she said confidently, 'and, um, minge?' She shrugged as if worried she'd taken a step too far as everyone laughed again. Louder this time.

'Flange!'

'Foofs!'

'Growlers,' That one ended me. I actually choked. As much as I wanted to melt into my plastic seat and never resurface, it was undeniably effective. Nothing bonds a room full of strangers quite like yelling 'muff' at nine in the morning. I felt I had heard all the possible names for vaginas out there. Imagine what I would say to Mum later when she'd ring and ask, 'How was your first day?' Oh well, see, the thing is, Mum, we talked about pussies, holes, cracks, bearded clams and the worst of the worst...cum dumpsters. Bloody hell. The last time I was involved in making a list like this was in A-Level geography where we listed mother nature's creations. I guess this was just a different perspective on that same brief. After all, whether it was your fandangle or your cha-cha slide, nature conjured it. Although, at that moment, I would have given anything to trade coochies and penis fly traps for ecosystems and global equilibrium...What had I done?

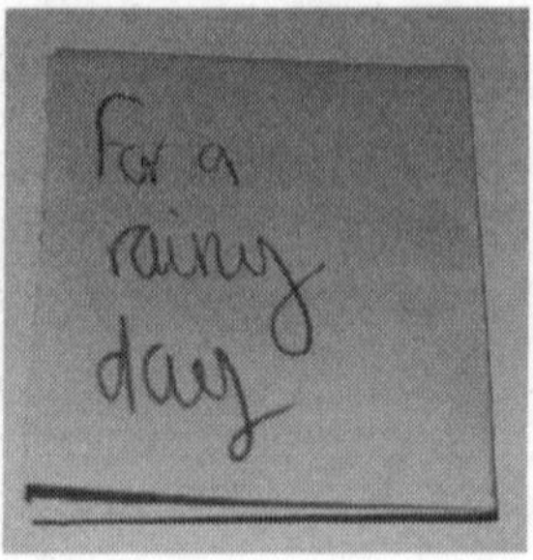
For a
rainy
day

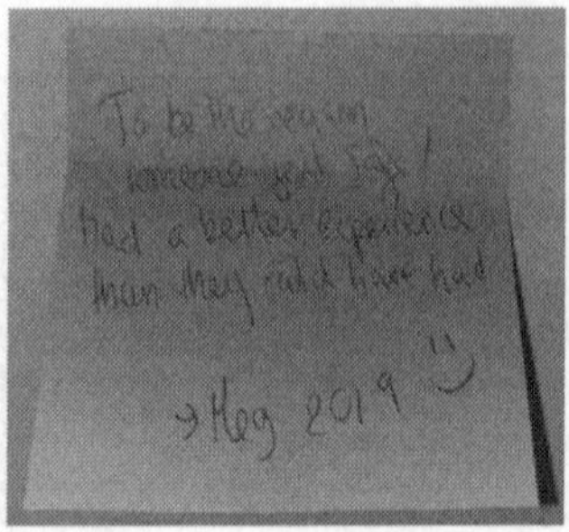
To be the reason
had a better experience
than Meg could have had
→ Meg 2019

*I took pictures of everything in case I lost it, including my little love note to future Meg

CHAPTER *Twenty*

BEA

'Well done, folks, we're done! Now get yourselves home!' Lynsey shouted after another research-heavy Friday. Everyone looked thrilled. After all, it was the weekend, and they were off to see their families or partners or just relax somewhere that didn't smell vaguely of mildew. Me? I was heading back to the cold, lime-green walls of uni halls. Homesickness was real, and I had it bad. I'd stopped eating properly.

I didn't smile like I used to either. I took regular trips home, they felt amazing, like someone had plugged my heart back in. But returning to Worcester? That stung more every time. The joy wore off by the time I reached the Severn Bridge. Maybe I wouldn't have felt so lonely if the girls in halls had clicked, but that didn't really happen. They had their own lives: partners to visit, people to FaceTime. I had Mum and Dad but even seeing them on a screen made me cry. And then I would cry because I *had* cried. The loneliness was like one of those Russian dolls, just sadness inside more sadness. I often beat myself up for feeling that way. I was aware of the world outside, how lucky I was, how much worse others had it. But I've learned (shoutout to Grandma, again): feelings don't care about context. They're still real. They still matter. They tell you when something's wrong and what you may need.

That night, I trudged back to Oak. The bile-coloured walls were as gross and judgmental as ever. I gave them the middle finger. Did it help? Not even a bit. But it felt like something. The others vanished into their rooms, and I flopped face-first onto my bed and cried. After half an hour, I tried to FaceTime Mum. No answer. Great. Cried some more. Eventually, my head started pounding. I peeled myself off the bed and kicked off my boots, catching my reflection in the mirror. Christ. I looked awful. Puffy eyes, blotchy skin, like I'd lost a fight with a bottle of vinegar. I was meant to be eighteen, fresh-faced, a beacon of youthful energy. Instead, I looked like a drained Capri-Sun. I often wondered what I'd become, and whether any of this was worth surviving on a banana, a few ginger nuts, and daily sobs whenever someone said 'family.'

My phone pinged with a text from Mum:

'Can I ring you about ten? Will look forward to it xx'

It was only half six. I tried to cry again, but nothing came. I was like a tiny desert. Emotionally arid. On that uplifting note, I dragged myself to the shower cubicles for a bit of resurrection. The uni bathrooms looked like they'd been inspired by an abandoned train station: grey, cold, and faintly traumatic. The showers were tiny. Only seven nozzles worked in the first cubicle, twelve in the second. Yes, I'd counted, boredom will do that to a person. Tonight, someone else had clearly done the maths too, and cubicle two was taken. So, I sulked into cubicle one, washed my hair twice, shaved everything, and dragged the whole ordeal out to forty minutes, partly because of the dribbling water pressure, but mostly because it meant less time crying in bed.

I returned to my room, hair wet, corridor silent, central heating still broken. Trembling like a Victorian orphan, I brushed my cold hair into a bun, every stroke pulsing in my skull. I looked at myself and laughed, that dry, slightly unhinged laugh that says, 'oh great, another personal low.' Collect the set. When would the highs come? When would I finally stop feeling like this? Then, at half eight, bored out of my skull, I opened my phone. Someone had messaged in the Sept 2019 uni group chat.

Bea: 'Hey girls, Friday night on my own isn't the best. Anyone around for a drink in Worcester area? Let me know if you fancy it. x'

My prayers. Answered. I replied within seconds: 'Yes please! Let me know where and I'll be there.'

Bea messaged me directly fifteen minutes later. No one else had responded. She lived on campus too, in a postgrad house with another girl from our cohort and two nurses. We arranged to meet at the student bar in twenty minutes. I got there in five.

The Student's Union was a big, open space with squishy chairs, TVs on the walls, and a second floor I'd never noticed before. For the first time since moving in, it felt vaguely... cosy. A petite, mousey-haired girl in a fluffy jumper spotted me and waved.

'Hey, is it Meg?' she smiled widely and adjusted a beaded bracelet on her wrist.

'That's me,' I smiled, taking the seat opposite her.

'Thanks so much for coming, I was getting so lonely in the house on my own.'

'Honestly? Same. I've been bloody miserable,' I said, half-laughing.

'Shall we grab a drink? You can fill me in.' She bought us two lemonades. I laughed, I thought I was the only one dodging alcohol at uni. And just like that, we talked. And talked. And talked. Bea was only a year older, she'd had a gap year living her best life, dressed as a Lego brick at Legoland. We covered it all: families, placements, gap year regrets, homesickness, favourite crisps, terrible ID photos. We laughed. We cried. We inhaled three lemonades and a Diet Coke to shake it up a little. At midnight, we called it a night. I couldn't believe we hadn't spoken before. I was so caught up in being lonely, I forgot to look up.

Oh, and I completely missed my FaceTime with Mum. But when I told her, she was over the moon. 'I'd rather you be out with someone than crying to me on a screen,' she said. Turns out Bea's mum had said the same. Neither of us knew it yet, but that was the start of something pretty beautiful.

CHAPTER
Twenty-One

PROBLEMATIC PLACEMENT

Life immediately improved the second Bea came into it, like someone dropped a glitter bomb in the middle of my stress-induced breakdown. We were inseparable: lectures, late-night takeaways, and existential crises, side by side. After a few weeks, the day was upon us to find out which practical placement we were heading to. Worcester uni had four placement options at the time:

'So, we want Worcester, right?' I asked Bea nervously. It was our longest placement of the three years, twelve weeks (instead of their initially proposed six).

'Yeah, it would be the shortest commute,' she said breezily from her bed, scrolling like this was any other Tuesday. Meanwhile, I was doing laps around her room like a caffeinated whippet.

'Meg, stand still a minute, it's refreshed. I've got Worcester, you?' I froze, thumb-jabbed my phone like a maniac, and squinted at the cursed text. I said the name of my placement allocation with no emotion, only shock. We now refer to this place and hospital trust as place X for too many reasons.

'Oh,' she said, peering over. 'But you don't even have your car here, do you?'

'No, because I'm a knob who's afraid of roundabouts, like a fish afraid of water,' I said with rising panic.

'You'd be fine Meg, I'm sure of it,' Bea said cooly. 'Come on Meg,' she prompted me. But that silence? That was the sound of my life collapsing into a rural black hole.

'Wait,' I eventually found some words. 'X is a fifty-minute drive away by car. Through country lanes. Not factoring in public transport,' I couldn't help thinking I was fucked as I felt my soul slowly leave the now empty cavity of my body.

The uni group chat was particularly active that afternoon, as everyone shared where they were allocated. Most people got the closest trust to where they lived, which was fair. However, they seemed to have forgotten about the university campus girls and chucked us at the end of the lists at random. Three joined me in X; one was Y, and the other got Worcester.

'Meg!' Bea clicked her fingers, laughing as she caught me in a staring competition with the wall.

'Sorry. I just don't know how I'm going to manage almost an hour's drive after a night shift,' I said, concerned.

'There will be a way,' Bea pulled my arm gently and guided me onto her bed. 'We will figure it out. It's for a couple of months, after which it will change again; I'm sure that's what they said.' She had a point. 'Maybe that's why they've done it, so you get your hospital placement closer for night shift work, as don't forget, this is community.'

'Bloody hell, I forgot it's not even at the hospital. It's *all over* X.' My soul returned to my body so I could have a moan.

'Meg, we will work it out, you'll get there, alright?' she kindly tried to reassure me.

'I just can't see past me crawling down a pitch-black country lane at 5 mph, white knuckling the wheel while a convoy of angry farmers curse my name. All because I'm trying to find someone's yurt. In the fog. With no signal.' I finally took a breath. We both sat, laughed at the thought, and went out for dinner to forget all about it.

After eating my grievances over X, the final week of theory at uni flew past and threw us all up and down with it like a bouncy ball in a washing machine. Here's how it all went down:

Monday 7th October 2019. Full day of lectures including the normal function of the placenta and later a shedload of research on breastfeeding. My breasts almost fell off themselves from the sheer boredom of the 'let down reflex'.

Tuesday 8th. Uniform fitting day. The uniform was a white tunic and navy trousers. *White*. For a midwifery degree. That's giving labour and birth a canvas to paint with blood, amniotic fluid and whatever else. Nevertheless, all thirty of us were cramped in a small room at the back of the campus with one guy running the fittings. When my name was called, I shuffled up like a contestant on the X-factor. The man radiated the energy of someone who ironed his socks for fun, looked me up and down with the intensity of a sniffer dog at Heathrow. No tape measure, no questions, just pure uncut judgement. He suddenly dove into the rail, rustled around like a raccoon in a wheelie bin, and dramatically produced... a size twenty-four. He held it up like it was the Holy Grail. Or maybe a warning.

'Next!' he barked, already moving on. I just stood there, stunned. I was a size fourteen a few minutes ago. I left the room a size twenty-four, a size four in dignity, and a size zero in will to live. Honestly, if I'd known humiliation was part of the uniform, I'd have brought a helmet.

Wednesday 9th. X emailed me a list of dos for student midwives and a longer list of don'ts, including not texting mentors on their days off, as she will likely need a break. At least the boundaries were clear I guess.

Thursday 10th. I bought a train pass for six weeks that cost me most of my student loan, coming in at £267.89. We weren't paid for any of our practical placement either. So, I was essentially paying the uni £9,000 a year to attend and nearly £300 to get there and back for six weeks. Goodbye, coffee. Goodbye, anything remotely fun for the foreseeable.

Friday 11th. I received an email saying we could claim back our travel money at some stage, although it was probably when I was forty and the NHS actually had some funding. I received another email telling me who my community supervisors were. I messaged them as instructed to give them my phone number, as it was, of course, completely acceptable for the midwives to text students whenever they wanted... Charlie sent me a friendly reply, while Joyce completely ignored my message. Naturally, I had more time rostered with Joyce. Of course I did.

Saturday 12th. A rare and beautiful day off, and I'm sure I spent most of it wondering how I'd become five dress sizes bigger and £300 down in the same week. A personal record.

Sunday 13th. My anxiety had anxiety. My thoughts were spiraling like a drunk figure skater: What if I forget everything? What if I accidentally call someones vagina a muff or a cooch? My heart was thumping like it had just downed three Red Bulls and wanted to fight God. Tomorrow, I'd officially become a student midwife. I didn't feel ready. I didn't feel professional. I didn't even feel like a competent adult. I felt like a badly disguised toddler who'd somehow conned her way into the NHS with a tunic a few sizes too big and a train ticket to nowhere. Whatever happened tomorrow, I'd be stepping into the weirdest, wildest chapter of my life. And probably someone's yurt.

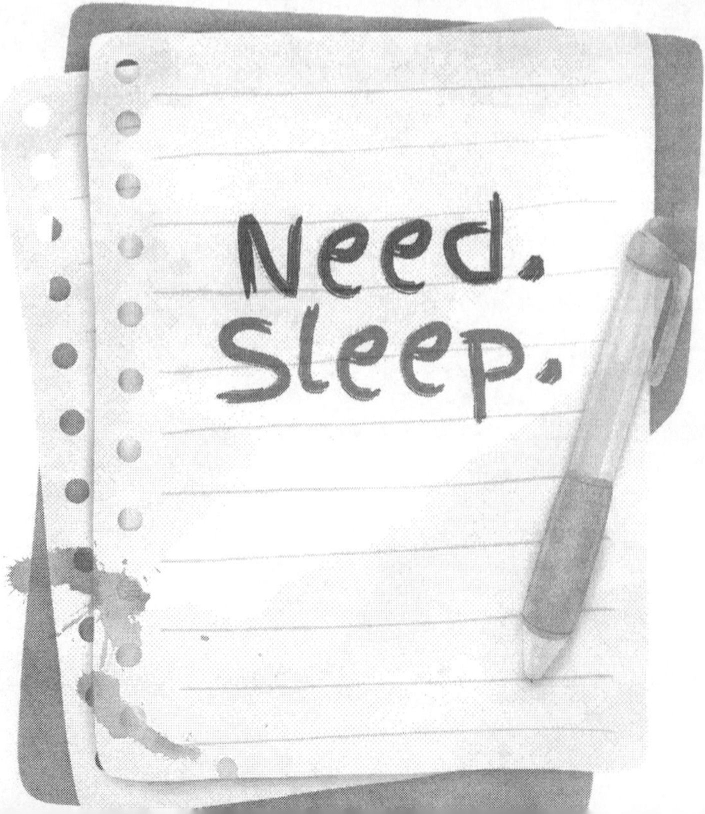
Need.
Sleep.

CHAPTER Twenty-Two

COMMUNITY CHAOS

October the fourteenth marked my first day of placement. Harriet, Amy and I walked fifteen minutes to Worcester train station. I felt like I was waddling, stuffed into a brand-new uniform that felt like a cardboard tent. By the time we reached the station, I could no longer feel my lower extremities; I was so cold. Meanwhile, Amy still declared herself the coldest whilst peeling off her hat, scarf and gloves. I think she my have forgotten that she'd moved to Worcester, not the Arctic Circle. A fifty-minute train journey later, three young student midwives stood on a random platform waiting for strangers to pick us up. What could possibly go wrong?

Amy was picked up first by a Range Rover and Harriet by someone who asked her what music she would like on route. I hung around and then a battered, grey Ford Focus hurtled around the corner and came to an abrupt halt. I knew instantly it was for me. The woman behind the wheel looked as tired as her car.

'Hi Joyce,' I said happily.

'Hello! You'd better get in then,' she declared. 'Hurry up!' She said, and I literally chucked myself into her passenger seat.

'Thank you for picking me up; I really appreciate it,' I said gratefully. She huffed. It was an excellent start.

'Ahh, it's alright,' she muttered. Was it, though? 'I just don't see why you guys don't drive. It makes it a longer morning for us getting ourselves stuck in traffic all the bloody time,' she explained the origin of her mood. I opened my mouth to respond but heard her voice instead.

'I have it every year, you know. Just for you all to drop out anyway,' she said sadly. I hadn't even shut the car door and already I was a statistical disappointment. Fantastic. Joyce started puffing up her fringe in the mirror whilst we waited in a traffic jam. She eventually turned to me and said, 'Sorry, Megan, it's not on you; we're all stretched at the moment,' she smiled, but frustration still lingered in her eyes. She may have realised she had been slightly abrupt for the first three minutes of knowing me.

'Oh, you bastard thing,' she spat at her handbrake as it struggled to be let off. The car jolted as it thrust forward.

'Is this your master plan, Joyce? To give me a little whiplash so I won't be asking for any more lifts?' I joked, clutching my neck as we whipped around another corner. She raised her eyebrows until they were lost in her bushy fringe, laughing, respecting a tickle of humour (thank God).

For the rest of the drive to Joyce's clinic, we chattered about the trials and tribulations of her work life and what I was signing myself up for. I found out she was happily married with three boys and looking forward to retiring for good in a few years. She'd already retired once but found herself drawn back to the job. I told her about my life so far, eighteen, fresh out of school with quite honestly no idea about the world outside of my own life. She seemed to value my honesty, accepting that I knew nothing.

We finally arrived at the small doctor's surgery just on the outskirts of X's main town centre. Joyce rolled up in the same parking space she had used for almost thirty years. Good job I didn't have my car, as I bet you, I'd have taken her space, and my career would have been over before it had even started. Anyway, Joyce hauled herself up and out of her car and slammed the door so hard her car shook. She ran her fingers through her fringe to buff it up, then proceeded to march to the back of her car. She thrust open her boot to reveal a literal mini market. There were orange juices, bottled water, crisps, peanuts, makeup and even a little hoover, just in case the urge to vacuum hit mid-appointment. She shoved it out of the way to reveal the baby scales and swung them over her shoulder almost taking me out in one clean swing.

'Shall I get this bag, Joyce?' I pointed towards a very full looking bag for life.

'No, no, that's my walking gear.' Of course it was. 'This,' she pointed down, 'is what we need, Megan.' She spoke through broken breath as she pulled out a mini suitcase. *A suitcase.* I couldn't help but laugh.

'Joyce,' I said as she stared at me, pretending as if this was your normal find. 'A flipping suitcase?' I picked it up and felt my arm strain. 'Where are you going? I had less when I moved in uni!' This was simply untrue, of course. I was the worst overpacker. I filled my poor dad's car up to the brim so much that he had to move his head between the toilet rolls to see out.

'Right,' Joyce laughed. 'Let's get in there,' she said as she led the way.

Once inside the clinic, room four had a low, bottled blue medical couch against one of the walls, a white sink in the corner opposite, a desk that Joyce sat on her blue spinny chair in front of and a counter just next to it. Joyce slammed her suitcase down on the floor and got on her hands and knees to unzip it. The left pocket had a funny little machine that looked like some sort of breathalyzer. What sort of woman was I about to meet? Sandwiched next to the breathalyzer were her blood pressure machine and several cuffs, urinalysis sticks, thermometers, a stethoscope, blood bottles, needles of different shapes and sizes, fat and thin syringes, plastic bags, blood/microbiology forms. You name it. Joyce had it. And if all went tits up, there was always the hoover. We set most of the contents of her suitcase across her room. I put some paper down on the couch whilst Joyce nearly threw her computer out of the window when she couldn't figure out how to log in. She eventually logged in and ran through the set-up for our day. We were going to see ten women in the clinic and then postnatal visits from half past four.

'Is every day booked up like this?' I asked, quite honestly surprised that there were so many pregnant women in X. I felt like I'd only seen about three pregnant people in my lifetime ever. Joyce looked at me, surprised that I even asked that...

'Always!' she said with a smile. 'Right, Chrissy is here. She's first up. Usually, we keep the first two hours free for new bookers, but Chrissy is one of my twenty-nine weekers who missed her appointment last week.' She took a quick breath. 'I did it all over the phone, but I need to take her blood quickly before our first official appointment arrives,' Joyce explained as she got her equipment ready.

'I'll go and get her?' I asked and headed for the door. Joyce nodded and I left for the main corridor. I walked past room two. A doctor smiled at me as I passed, an unfamiliar but welcome surprise. Being on the other side of a doctor's surgery was a strange feeling. Most doctors didn't even smile at me when I went in for appointments. Was it my new role? I felt important for a moment. I poked my head into the waiting room and called Chrissy to the door. A slim woman with a little bump protruding from her black jacket came forward. She had her hair slicked back and tied in a bun at the back of her head, and she had big golden loop earrings. I introduced myself and started to lead her to room four. Although I saw a different doctor this time. I looked up and found the number eight. Confused, I turned around, panicking that this woman would think I was useless, and tried to figure out where I went so wrong. Although Chrissy was already five steps ahead of me; she grabbed my wrist, spun me around and took me the right way to room four.

'It's a weird system, love. Don't worry about it. Do it a few times, and you'll be fine,' she said kindly. I felt my cheeks burn as I smiled back in embarrassment, and my newfound importance disappeared as quickly as it came.

'Alright, Joyce?' Chrissy threw out as she flung the door open.

'Chrissy, come in, come in,' Joyce didn't even turn her head away from her computer screen. I shuffled in after her. 'So, how are you?' Joyce asked.

'I'm alrigh, I think,' Chrissy replied as she scratched her lower bump.

'You think?' Joyce questioned over her thick glasses frame.

'Well, I've got a funny smell from down there at the moment. Never happened with my last,' Chrissy explained as it turned out she was itching her vagina, not her bump. Wonderful.

'Best start with your urine sample!' Joyce took the sample and passed it to me to dip. As instructed, I put the urinalysis stick* in the sweet, putrid-smelling urine, and the stick glowed like a city skyline. I wafted it in front of Joyce's face.

'Most likely a UTI,' Joyce scuffed and put her head in her suitcase to retrieve a sample bottle.

'Can you look tho Joyce?' Chrissy asked as she stood up, lifted her dress and sat on the couch.

'It's only supposed to be your bloods today, not whatever you've got going on down there!' Joyce laughed, they clearly had a solid relationship as Chrissy laughed and gave her a specific look. 'Right, let's have a quick look then,' Joyce tutted as she plucked some blue examination gloves from her box.

'Is it okay with you, Chrissy, if I stay with Joyce while she has a look?' I asked Chrissy sensitively.

'Course, love. You got to learn somewhere, haven't you?' She flashed me a smile. I thanked her and helped her adjust herself on the couch.

'Right en,' Chrissy struggled as she got her underwear off. 'Catch!' She launched them at me. I missed and witnessed the pair of sodden knickers land on the floor with a wet slap. Joyce put her head in her hand whilst Chrissy laughed so hard that her skin lifted and hid her little blue eyes beneath it. Her mouth was wide open and revealed that her front tooth was flying solo in there. I quickly put on a pair of blue gloves and retrieved the item from the floor, and the smell hit me. I stood there with them in my hands, and I realised I had no idea where I was going to put them. I couldn't just sling them in her little green handbag. Imagine when she opened that later on... Joyce just watched me pivot, trying to figure out where to put them for her.

'Chuck em in my coat pocket, love, unless you have a bag or sommet Joyce?' Chrissy was lying down on the couch now, parting her labia for Joyce to look at as easily as it was to open your curtains in the morning. I don't know if Joyce or I got the worst deal at that moment.

'Grab a red blood form, Meg; you can seal them in there,' Joyce said through pursed lips. It looked like the smell had gotten to her nose, too; she wasn't laughing anymore. 'Grab me a blue one as well Meg, we're gonna need something to go off to micro from you Chrissy. Likely an infection of some sort,' Joyce said as she helped her get off the couch. After a lengthy discussion of signs and symptoms, Joyce took Chrissy's bloods, which was also weird to witness. The blood was pouring into the bottles as Joyce held the needle still in her vein in her arm. This did not happen on the plastic arms at uni; 'blood flow' was slow, and you had to put the needle so far in it looked as if it would come out the other end. Definitely not the same in reality, Joyce had barely scratched the surface of her skin.

'Right,' Joyce huffed at the computer, 'I'll let you know what happens with the urine and bloods. If you can book in with the GP, you'll probably beat this sample as it takes a few days,' Joyce advised Chrissy honestly. You've got your next appointment with me in the books. If there are any problems, call me, or, if it's urgent, ring triage, yes?' Joyce demanded confirmation.

'Yes, boss!' Chrissy stood up and saluted Joyce. 'I know the drill innit. Thanks Joyce, you always sort me out. And you, Meg, thanks for dealing with them, I wouldn't have.' She took her knickers back out of my hands. I was so delighted that I hadn't screwed up entirely and to be thanked that I panicked and said, 'Was a pleasure!' What a weird choice of words. Joyce's face was screwed up, telling me she thought exactly the same.

After Chrissy and her knickers left, we were running late. Joyce stormed through the two booking appointments that had been scheduled for the rest of the morning. Both ladies we met were under twelve weeks pregnant, and it was their first appointment with a midwife. The amount of information Joyce had covered, the samples she took, the forms she filled in, the referrals she made and the responsibility she had to ensure it was all done, blew my mind. I quickly realised you needed that two-hour block as a booking appointment was like speed-dating your entire life history, with added urine. We covered medical history, problems with themselves, their partner and then both families (maybe we'd ask about the dog next time), mental health, and social issues. Based on the answers, it triggered different referrals; for example, one lady had a Body Mass Index (BMI) of fifty-five, so she had a referral for a diabetic screen, a different dose of folic acid and something else as well. How did she know to make those adjustments for a woman she'd only just met? To me, as a brand-new student midwife, it was equal parts intimidating and impressive.

Following the two new 'bookers' as Joyce described them, we had half an hour appointment slots from this point. They were all ladies Joyce had met before, and this helped massively. A lady called Akaiya blew a fourteen on the breathalyser, which I assumed wasn't good as it flashed red aggressively. Turned out it was a carbon monoxide monitor and indicated Akaiya was likely smoking more than her admitted one cigarette a day. One lady, Karen, was thirty-eight weeks pregnant with her first baby and asked if she could use cooking oil instead of lavender oil on her perineum to help it stretch for labour? Joyce said no. Another woman, Alison, was thirty-three weeks pregnant with twins and asked if twins were always born on the same day. Joyce explained that it would only happen if one was born at the last minute of the day and the next after midnight. It's not like one would come out and leave the other behind for a few years. One woman, Lisa, had a blood pressure reading of 184/112. And considering the normal parameters were 110-140/60-90, Joyce sent her to the hospital almost as quickly as she had taken that reading. It was jam-packed, and the clock read quarter-past five before we knew it. We were supposed to finish at half-part four, but I guess we went on for a lot longer as I was asking lots of questions at the end of appointments, to which Joyce usually had long answers. She was a wealth of knowledge, and I had already learnt so much.

'Thankfully, we don't have any postnatal visits anymore tonight, Meg,' Joyce said with relief as she slid lower down her blue chair. 'They've been readmitted via triage. What a day. What did you think?' She asked curiously.

'I have no words, Joyce, haha,' I said truthfully, not knowing where to begin.

'Well done. You did well. You have a nice way with the women, and that's important.' She smiled. 'I'll see you for more of the same tomorrow, yes?' she said with authority.

'Ahh, thanks, Joyce. Although I couldn't help but feel pretty useless today,' I added, trying to conceal the uneasiness. I was overwhelmed, to say the least.

'You'll get there. Learn to worry about one thing at a time,' Joyce reassured me. With that, we packed away her suitcase and headed out of the room through the empty surgery and back to Joyce's knackered car. I was beginning to understand how her car was feeling after all.

*The art of poking a stick in pee and pretending its high science. Midwives are obsessed with it, and for good reason. It can pick up protein (this is your informal pre-eclampsia warning), sugar (hi, gestational diabetes), blood (another can of conditions) and all sorts else. It's like a rainbow of detection. National guidance has made it compulsory for urinalysis to be performed at every antenatal contact as an integral part of antenatal care.

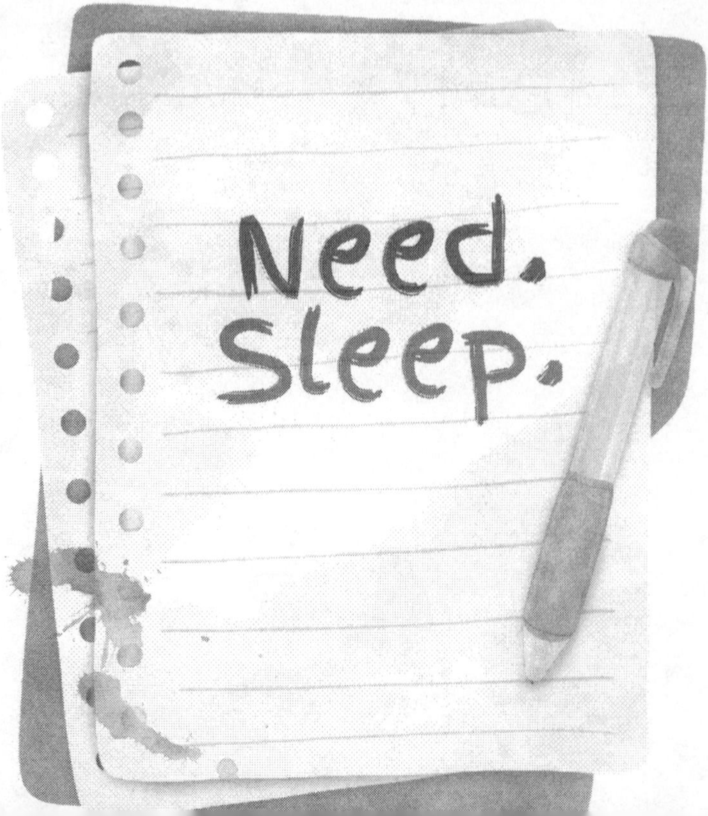
Need.
Sleep.

CHAPTER
Twenty-Three

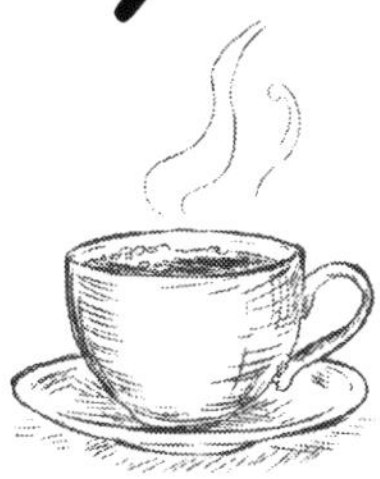

JACK AND JOYCE DOWN COUNTRY LANES

By week five of placement, the leaves had gone from auburn to brown, and it wasn't only the seasons that were changing. I'd gone from clueless to slightly less clueless at least. Joyce, and the chaos of community midwifery had become my compass, whether I liked it or not. Even so, I gained insight into both lower and higher-risk care pathways and life beyond being eighteen. I witnessed one extreme to the next; for example, one time, we visited a giant country house to do a postnatal check where the baby actually had his own bathroom already (at the grand age of three days old). In contrast, the next visit was to a woman who told us she had used the ready-to-use formula milk almost like squash, adding water to it to make it last longer, which was unfortunately seriously unsafe to do so. She cried over affording it, and I felt like I wanted to buy her formula myself, as we broke the news to her. Another long and hard lesson was the art of learning to care professionally and not personally, something that wouldn't be mastered overnight.

Amongst the varied social demographics, I had also gotten stuck in with too many clinical skills; I had a go at abdominal palpation, where midwives somehow figured out exactly where the baby was lying within the cushioned uterus. Most times I had a go, it felt like all limbs and no idea, but apparently, that also came in time. I was so pleased to have successfully taken someone's blood the other week, so much so that I forgot to take the tourniquet off when I withdrew the needle, causing blood to spray everywhere, including all over me, the woman and the floor. What a knob. I had a little notebook to write useful bits of info such as *'take the tourniquet off!!!!!'* Which I scribbled underneath the title *'venepuncture'*. Whether it was auscultating the fetal heart rate (FHR) or measuring the growing bump, I enjoyed being part of something so essential and fundamental, yet it was ever-changing. New evidence and, subsequently, new guidelines were always critically questioned, and recommendations for practice were interchangeable. A truly mind-blowing industry to be a part of.

On the fifth of November, Joyce and I had a very hectic clinic day, working from eight until four. This time we had a home visit to go to in the middle of Welsh territory.

'Meg, I've had enough of this,' Joyce sat behind her steering wheel and complained about the house we were supposed to be visiting. Joyce jabbed at the satnav like it owed her money.

'It won't pick it up, the damn thin, she spat at 'the machine', as she called it. The screen flashed between 'no route found' and what suspiciously looked like a body of water. Assuming our next patient wasn't living on the rocks with the crew of Finding Nemo, I reached for her ancient road map instead. It smelled like the 1970s and had more creases than her forehead. To make it slightly worse, the sun was just setting, which meant the tiny, black letters on the map only got harder to decipher.

'Beautiful sky though Joyce, look!' I tried to divert her rage to the beautifully sinking sun for a moment.

'We'll lose the damn sun in a minute!' She snapped back. I almost got my little notebook out to write *'Never interrupt a midwives rage'* but thought better of it.

Anyway, after twenty-five minutes of driving, we meandered through country lanes, where the ground naturally got a little rougher. The dips were deeper, and the inclines were steeper. However, apparently no match for Joyce. She braced herself, pushed her head forward, squinted and slammed her foot to the accelerator, which I'm sure hit the floor and literally took us over the treacherous lanes in a flash. I felt the water that I had just had a sip of a few moments ago being thrown against the sides of my stomach. We finally reached a big wooden gate where Joyce came to an abrupt stop. I couldn't help but shoot her a look after that performance.

'What!' Joyce responded. 'The quicker we get here, the quicker we're outta here,' she added matter-of-factly. The wave of nausea inhibited my ability to reply, instead, I looked at our surroundings out of the window. It seemed between us and the house there was a field, a few ditches and a hill that we needed to navigate, in the dark, in the winter. I eventually got out of the car, shivering as the bitter wind caught my back and joined Joyce at the back of her car. As our usual protocol, we hauled bits of her kit between us.

'Right, let's go,' Joyce tightened the straps of the baby scales bag over both her shoulders. I nodded and walked alongside her. We crossed a little path and opened a wooden gate to a field of sheep; it was like we were visiting Mary and her little lambs.

'They all say community is easy Meg,' she huffed, 'I'd love to see how delivery suite would enjoy this,' Joyce exclaimed as she stared up at the hill we needed to climb to get to the farmhouse.

'I can't even see that well Joyce!' I started putting one foot after the other to ensure the ground was stable before weight bearing on it.

'Well, you'll have to open your eyes more!' Joyce adjusted her wellies and charged straight past me up the hill with her fringe leading the way. Outrun by a fifty-five-year-old. Brilliant.

Paved with sandy-coloured stone, the house was about twice the size of mine, so it was no wonder it needed its own lane, hill, and field. The doorway was dimly lit by two small light bulbs, so, I, with the miscellaneous equipment bag and Joyce, with the baby scales, headed over and gave the grand-looking knocker a knock. A dog with a high-pitched bark started to shout at us, alerting their very tired owner. Elizabeth opened the door and had more bags under her eyes than Joyce and I had on our backs. She apologised for her poodle, Darcie and led us across her wide, unperturbed hallway, which was decorated with many framed pictures of herself and her husband. Darcie ran ahead excitedly to the living room where the baby, Theodore, was crying in his Moses basket. Elizabeth took a seat in the chair and dropped her head into her hands; the kind of silent collapse only sleep deprivation can cause. It hit me then, I was eighteen, barely able to look after myself, and here I was, pretending to know how to help this woman recover from major surgery while raising a brand-new human. Whilst I settled young Theo, Joyce made Elizabeth a cup of tea and fielded the questions I couldn't answer. The half-an-hour slot had come to an end, and although I felt the biggest sense of imposter syndrome, we left a calmer Elizabeth and Theo for the night ahead, so I took it as a win. It was coming up to six o'clock by the time we left, and it was as if someone had switched the stars off. It was pitch black. If I thought I couldn't see before, I could barely make out Joyce's figure in front of me. We both got to the bottom of the hill where the car was, but the darkness was making the line between the ground and the now well-concealed ditch very difficult.

'Now, watch yourself!' Joyce snapped as I watched my right foot slip a few inches underneath me. 'You nearly tripped then; that's the last thing I need for you to do something stupid down a mudslide!' She barked. I wasn't planning on wrestling nature. However, it seemed that nature had its own ideas of wrestling Joyce, and with that, she slipped on what looked and smelt like some sort of poo and flew into a blur of blue down the other side of the car, down quite a deep ditch.

'Fuck,' I said as I lost sight of my mentor. Bigger fuck, she was thirty-seven years older than me, and that slope posed a danger to me, let alone Joyce and her self-proclaimed dodgy back. Biggest fuck yet, she was my ticket back home, so leaving her to tend the sheep just wasn't an option.

'Joyce!' I shouted loudly into the darkness. 'Joyce, are you okay?' I repeated.

'I'm-kay,' she stuttered. 'Bruised, no doubt, but I'm okay. Now get your arse down here!' Taking her sarcasm as a sign, she was fine, I couldn't help myself and shouted back.

'What have you done that for? That was pretty stupid; it's all I needed!' I winced at the blank environment and held my breath as I waited for her response.

'Very funny!' Her voice boomed, and we both burst into laughter. I flicked my phone torch on and saw her just getting up from the ground. To be fair, you could see that fringe from a mile away and that was without the torch. The best bit was that she instructed me to stay put as she lobbed her blood pressure machine up the hill for me to catch, and thank God I did as,

'It's precious that mind,' she said after launching it up towards me. It was like watching a live remake of Jack and Jill, except I certainly did not go tumbling after; I just stood there trying to catch expensive equipment. I had visions of lessons to put into my little notebook.

- *Take tourniquet OFF.*
- *Never interrupt Joyce mid-rage.*

- *Mud is NOT sterile or to be taken lightly in the winter.*

'I knew I should have kept the scales. Like I always do,' Joyce muttered as she clambered her way back up the landslide. When she was finally on the same elevation level as me, I saw that her hair was sticking out edgeways, and the mud discoloured her blues so much so that she said she looked the same once when she finished a shift with a lady with explosive diarrhoea. In labour. I shuddered at the thought of a shit-stained Joyce and also what was lying ahead of me as we headed for the car. I turned my attention back to the current situation, Joyce with wild hair, muddy blues, and the faint smell of something unholy and thought, 'Yep. This is it. This is the dream.'

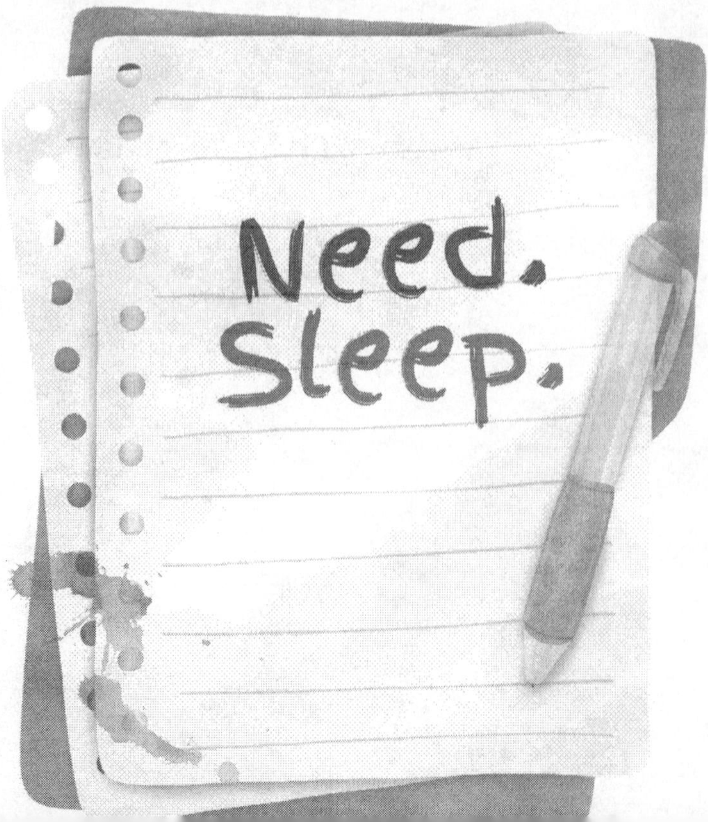
Need.
Sleep.

CHAPTER Twenty-Four

HAPPY HOME-BIRTHDAY

Twelve weeks into my community placement in X, and uni already felt like a distant dream. This was the real deal; blood, babies, and all things bonkers. I arrived at the community office to meet Joyce on my last day of first-year placement, the next time I'd be in the community would be year three. The thought made me feel slightly sick. X's community office was sandwiched between Delivery Suite and Maternity Ward. The bridge between them both. It was a tiny office; the wall on the right-hand side was stacked floor to ceiling with case notes. The left had one long continuous desk. Boxes of all sorts were stuffed underneath. I watched paper forms fluttering from the warm air stream propelled by the fan in the corner. Two midwives I didn't recognise were in this morning. Sighing and typing alternatively.

'Hiya,' I said as I entered. One ignored me, and the other offered a smile but nothing more. I sat awkwardly on the end of a stool behind the whirring fan.

'Who are you here for?' The smiley one asked.

'Joyce,' I said straight away.

'Lovely, okay,' she said, returning to her screen. The other midwife looked up to observe the conversation that had disturbed her and turned back to her screen. Joyce was often late, so I whipped my phone out for a few minutes, hoping I wouldn't sit there awkwardly for too long. However, the minutes turned into twenty minutes with no text, and I got worried. The midwife who smiled at me had left ten minutes before, and just the one who ignored me remained. She was still furiously typing and huffing.

'Excuse me?' I awkwardly asked, approaching her from the side. Nothing.

'I. Um. Excuse me,' I squeaked.

'Talking to me, are you?' She said flatly. Considering she was the only midwife in the office, I hoped it was her I was talking to.

'Yes, sorry, I'm wondering if you know if Joyce is coming by any chance? I'm supposed to be with her today, and it's not like her to be this late.' I asked nervously.

'Joyce's off sick,' she said plainly. Brilliant. I had no idea. I sat there for half an hour, and she knew I was waiting for a midwife who would never turn up.

'Right, okay, that's frustrating; I've sat here since nine,' I said, flatter than usual. No reply again, of course. Awkwardly, I returned to sitting on the stool and contemplated what to do next.

Suddenly, a different midwife flew through the door. She was slight but had energy twice her size. She knocked over the other midwife's bag off the desk. I had to try and suppress a smile.

'Sorry, love,' she said, bending down to retrieve it. When she had no response, she flicked her eyebrows up at me. At least I wasn't alone. Her name was Sarah, and she had a day of visits off the grid today. When I said I was supposed to be with Joyce, I was hoping she'd offer to have me.

'Ahh, I've got Harriet in the car waiting for me. Sorry, love,' she said sincerely. Lucky Harriet. God damn it. Before I got the chance to reply, her phone started ringing. She almost disappeared in her bag, trying to find it. The other midwife scowled at the noise she was making. If she was upset about this, then she was in for a lot worse when Sarah was chatting on the phone. I'm pretty sure Harriet would have heard the conversation from outside.

'Ahh dear, okay, that is quite the situation,' Sarah said.

'Multip?' She nodded as she wrote many things on the back of an Asda receipt.

'We will have to send Letitia. There's no other option due to sickness,' she said, looking towards the other midwife in the room. The other midwife, Letitia, looked as though someone had just died at this point. Oh dear. I was glad to be spectating.

'My student and I have visits out as far as Abergavenny, so we can take Letitia's visits for sure and do hers on route,' Sarah confirmed. Letitia stared blankly at her.

'We do have a student here, actually, supposed to be with Joyce, but of course, she isn't here today,' Sarah said, looking over her shoulder at me. She covered the bottom of the phone and mouthed, 'Do you want a home birth?' I nodded instinctively and felt the adrenaline tingle through my chest. I'd not seen a birth yet and didn't think I would until the hospital placement, as the midwives had said there were no planned home births for the weeks I was in the community.

'Kay then, take care, yes, I will, okay, bye-bye,' Sarah hollered.

'Right then, is it Megan? You are off to a homebirth with Letitia!' Her grin widened while mine faltered. Letitia's reaction exceeded mine; she slammed her diary on the desk, which caused the mouse to fly off and dangle down in her way as she got up and fought her way past it. She picked up a bag from under the desk and muttered words that sounded awfully like 'fuck's sake' and 'typical' under her breath before pausing in the doorway. Maybe she was under the thumb of burnout? Still processing a poor event? Either way, her manner was quite unnerving.

'Are you coming or what?' She shot at me. I scrambled off my feet and waved bye to an apologetic-looking Sarah. That initial excitement was so short-lived and just as quickly replaced by dread.

The drive to the woman's address was long, but the drive felt longer with Letitia. I asked a few questions, to which Letitia replied with the relevant information but nothing more than that. It was going to be my first witness. As a student midwife, it was required by the Nursing and Midwifery Council (NMC), to witness five uncomplicated, spontaneous vaginal births before being hands-on. Of course, I hadn't even met a labouring woman, let alone seen a birth. Letitia was happier when she found out I was 'only witnessing' and, therefore, 'wouldn't be in the way'. That was something, at least. Although I felt so insignificant, as I sat next to her. We arrived at the property after a very bumpy lane. Letitia's tightly scraped ponytail loosened slightly as rocks pinged underneath the tyres. I considered faking car sickness just to be sent home, but with no means for transport home, this was it. The house was huge, a crimson-coloured barn conversion by the looks.

'So,' Letitia spat as she flung her seatbelt off. 'You're going to respect the birthplace. You're going to sit at the back of the room on the floor, watch, don't speak, and try not to pass out,' she said with admonition. Unbelievable. I couldn't actually comprehend what I was being asked of and how it was being asked of me. I felt like a total nuisance. The excitement I felt kept trying to leap through, but fear weighed it down.

I followed Letitia into the woman's house and into the living room. The woman was on all fours and breathing through a forceful contraction.

'Hi Letitia,' another midwife, Lucy, welcomed her. 'And is it, Megan?' she said warmly. Thank God, a nice midwife. Just a shame I wasn't here with Joyce instead of Letitia.

'Megan's only witnessing,' Letitia hissed.

'First year, Meg?' Lucy asked me kindly whilst shooting a look towards Letitia.

'Yes, first year, first placement, and hopefully first witness,' I said with the first genuine smile since I met Sarah back at the hospital. Lucy beamed excitedly for me, and she got into the details of Jody's situation.

'Jody. Forty weeks and one day. Gravida two, para one (G2, P1)*. Uncomplicated, midwife-led care,' Lucy paused to help Jody through another mighty contraction that took over her body. She rocked with the pain, but eventually, it subsided, and I introduced myself to her, ignoring Letitia's previous desire for my silence.

Jody was chatty between contractions, which was lovely as I managed to build a good rapport with her and her partner, Steve. They already had a little boy to whom they wanted to introduce their new baby by the end of his school day. Tough gig that. Apparently, not for a multip, though. Lucy taught me that a rule of thumb is second labours are generally quicker than the first as the body has done it before. A little like muscle memory.

A couple of hours went on, and I was chuffed that Jody let me get stuck in, and Lucy supported me in doing it despite Letitia's annoyance. I got going with some observations (blood pressure, pulse, oxygen saturation, temperature, respiratory rate) when needed. Jody was happy for me to have a go at auscultating the baby's heart rate too. We needed to do this every fifteen minutes in established labour and every five minutes in the second stage (full cervical dilatation/pushing stage). I transferred my community skills of counting the rate for a minute to establish a baseline. You can tell an awful lot by a baby's heart rate; however, what is important and equally quite scary to remember is that you are confirming fetal wellbeing at that moment, hence the importance of frequent auscultation and escalating any signs of concern immediately.

The normal parameters for a baby's heart rate to sit at is between 110 and 160 beats per minute. Jody's baby was sitting at around 135 bpm. Fluctuations within the baseline are also important. An increase in heart rate for a short period is called an acceleration and is often associated with fetal movements and wellbeing. However, the reverse is classed as a deceleration and another topic altogether. There's much more to decelerations than I knew then, but at the time, all I understood was: decels = possible distress. Escalate fast. Again, there is much more to this than meets the eye, but as a first year on first placement, this is generally what I needed to know.

Over the next few hours, Jody's body progressed beautifully, and by ten o'clock, she had started pushing. Lucy somewhat agreed with Letitia in the sense of having a seat behind the midwives whilst she birthed her baby, but she wanted me to have the chance to soak it in, observe, and enjoy my first witness. A much nicer rationale than Letitia's, that was for sure. So, I knelt on my knees at their fireplace and watched as Jody pushed, and slowly but surely, the top of the baby's head (vertex) was visible.

After a few minutes, the vertex was advancing well, and Lucy used a warm pad to support Jody's perineum as her baby's head edged its way into the world.

'Pant now, Jody, don't push,' Lucy instructed softly; Jody puffed and panted away the pain rather than pushing as her baby crowned.

'Stingy bit now, little push,' Lucy encouraged her. I watched as the baby's forehead emerged, quickly followed by the appearance of two little eyebrows.

'I can see up to baby's nose now, Jody; you are doing a wonderful job,' Lucy beamed. Letitia was busy writing down the times of events. Baby's chin eventually emerged, and it was strange yet amazing to see a baby's head resting between their mum's legs. It was incredible as I watched the baby turn their head to the right. I know this movement now as restitution, which is the art of baby moving their shoulders underneath the pubic bone.

If restitution isn't seen, we get anxious for shoulder dystocia where, essentially, the baby's shoulders haven't been able to move under the pubic arch and are, therefore, stuck. This is one of life's scariest emergencies and something to discuss later on.

But for this day, and for Jody, her baby restituted as expected and her baby even twitched their nose and flickered their eyelids as they were ready for their life to begin.

'One more contraction, one more push, Jody, and we will have your baby,' Lucy said happily. Jody smiled to Steve who was holding both of her hands as we all awaited the final contraction.

'Here we go!' Jody exclaimed, and with that, baby's shoulders and body came flying into the word. Lucy gave the baby a rub with a towel and passed them up to Mum.

'Is it a boy?' Steve asked immediately, and their baby cried in response. Lucy helped to lift the baby so both parents could see.

'A little girl, Steve!' Jody exhaled. A beautiful baby girl was looking around her living room as if it was where she'd always been. What a thing to watch! I felt a strong emotion tickle my eyes, but nothing further as I focused on Jody's blood loss instead.

Although it seemed like a lot of blood at the moment, Jody lost a perfectly normal amount in the end, and her placenta came out with ease around twenty minutes later. Lucy checked her perineum for tears, but there were none. Lucy said it may have had a good deal to do with Jody breathing her baby out in a controlled way, not quickly. I didn't think this could have gone better for Jody. And as for baby Enid, as we came to know her, it was as if she had read the breastfeeding manual before coming out. I supported Jody to latch her to the breast, but she didn't need any more than that. So, we cleaned, wrote a lot of documentation, and accepted a cup of tea from Steve before we left. Conveniently, we left around three o'clock, just in time for Steve to do the school run as if nothing had ever happened. I was on an all-time high; the positive adrenaline pumping through my veins was so much that even Letitia couldn't knock it. The birth buzz, as we call it, lasted right until the following morning, and I realised I was feeling optimistic about my choice at the present time and enjoyed the moment for all it was worth. To my surprise, Letitia was much tamer on the journey home, and she even gave me a wry smile when I thanked her for having me, as we all knew how much it aggrieved her. I guess things weren't all that bad after all.

* Gravida is the total number of pregnancies a person has had (including the current one). Parity (para for short) refers to the number of births. Losses make things a little trickier: for example, someone with one live child and two miscarriages is recorded as G3, P1+2. Losses before 24 weeks (the legal threshold of viability) are counted in the '+' number. Stillbirths (losses after 24 weeks) are included in parity, so a person with one stillbirth and two live babies would be G3, P3.

CHAPTER Twenty-Five

FATEFUL FRUIT PASTILLES

After that first placement, I spent a few more weeks at uni, where theory block put a massive distance between me and placement life, and despite questionable mentors, I missed it. Only two others and I were lucky enough to attend a home birth; I wouldn't forget Jody, Steve, and baby Enid in a hurry. By mid-December, we had submitted two essays and a supporting presentation. Although, in my group, one of the students, Theresa, turned her allocated five minutes into twenty, the timer went off, and the other four of us didn't get a chance to say our piece. A low pass was still a pass, I guess.

I finally moved on when we were unleashed for the Christmas break, where I quickly discovered one of my favourite feelings was arriving home for Christmas 2019. You'd have thought I'd been away overseas or something about how much I radiated happiness when I arrived. I contacted an old friend from school, but not R, S or Tommy. R and I message back and forth every now and then, checking in and updating each other; he was studying business at Uni in Bangor (at least one of us made it there), he also had a long-term girlfriend, Serena, and he was happy, therefore, so was I. On the other hand, last both R and I heard, S dropped out of Cardiff uni, where he was studying art and went rogue, where nobody seemed to know what he was up to. On the other hand, Tommy promised he'd meet for coffee next time he was home; the last Facebook update showed him open-water swimming in Finland, I guess some things never change.

One of my oldest friends, Lyssa, made up for what she lacked in height with her energy; she was always on top of the world and often raised me with her. She helped me that once in year eight when I sat underneath a tree and cried after flinging my leggings off in the middle of a summer run. Rough times. Anyway, Lyssa and I remained close friends despite growing up to be polar opposites. For example, I was too afraid to breach any rules, whereas Lyssa had to be reminded what the definition of a rule was. Lyssa loved a drink at a party, but I'd ask her where she kept her squash. Nevertheless, we accepted and embraced each other exactly as we were and gained a lot from each other as a result.

'I reckon we go Cardiff, big nite out, yuh?' This was the text I received at three-forty am on a Tuesday morning. I did not even have to look at the name of the text from which it originated, but I knew who it was from. Although I wasn't sure if I could handle drink, I had tried it on New Year's Eve with my family last year, but it only gave me a splitting headache and opened the gates to the sad sphere of my brain which questioned my existence and sent me into a panic. Plus, clubs, crowds and autism mixed worse than any alcohol concoctions could. So, although I always appreciated her invites to her big nights, I said no. But I did understand one thing, different people enjoy different things and friendships, if anything, are about compromise. Plus, I missed her. So, after a year of declining her wild invitations, I finally said yes. It was time to face the inevitable. Clubbing. With Lyssa.

'No way, Meg. Never thought you actually say yeh!' She shouted down the phone.

'Haha, I need to see you; it's been way too long,' I said as I turned the volume down on my car.

'Great, you can come mine to get dressed, pres then we hit Prizm! I've booked our entry tickets. Quids in, yeah?' She finally took a breath.

'Quids in?' I put both hands on the wheel in anticipation.

'Come on. One quid to get in, Meg?' She said, astonished. I couldn't decide whether that news was good as I wouldn't be losing anything by going or bad as it must be shit to cost a quid for entry. Regardless, I agreed anyway. It was about spending time with Lyssa this time. Nothing else really mattered to me, at least it didn't when I was in the safety of my car.

The day quickly rolled around. I met Lyssa at the entrance to her uni quarters. She was studying comedy in Cardiff. She didn't need it, though; she was hysterical without even trying. She came hurtling down her front steps with neon pink rollers scattered amongst her thick brown hair. She had a bright blue dressing gown on with yellow sliders. I ran over to her and wrapped my arms around her.

'Watch the tan, though, Meg,' she said as she brushed me off her. Although I ended up brushing her off, quite literally, as I looked down at my white top, I found little molecules of fake tan sitting on the material that was not quite sunken yet. I didn't care, so I gave her a bottle of her favourite vodka and headed into her uni digs. She led me through the remains of their kitchen (this wasn't the first party her house had seen that week) and up to her room. Bright pink curtains and big bright lightbulbs shone on the outskirts of her mirror. I flopped on her bed and talked for an hour before I moved to get remotely ready.

'What the fuck is that?' Lyssa asked me in shock as I pulled up my tights.

'What do you mean?' I said while I checked my tights for any holes.

'You're wearing tights. To a club?' she said, her face distorted. 'And what is this all about?' She plucked my turtleneck jumper. 'You're not going to a convent, Meg,' she roared, laughing.

'The cheek!' I smacked her with the sleeve of my turtleneck jumper.

'You're never going to pull looking like that; the only bit of your skin I can see is your face. I'm not going out with you looking like that,' she said in hysterics, but I knew she was also damn serious. As a result, Lyssa brought out a bright pink dress which cinched her body in all the right places. She had heels on, and even though they left marks a few inches deep on her carpet, she was ready to face the world. In all fairness, she was right; I looked like I was about to attend a court hearing and had the facial expressions to match.

Moments later, she staggered to her wardrobe and disappeared into it. Unlike Narnia, I wasn't willing to go in after her. Instead, I sat on the edge of her bed and let out intermittent bouts of nervous laughter. The scary reality was that the outfit I had brought was the nicest I had owned. Lyssa finally emerged and tried to catch her breath. She threw a few items at me and raised her eyebrows instructively to say get them on!

'Oh fu-' I said worriedly to the mirror and felt the colour drain from my face. I looked like a glitzy cowgirl prostitute. I had black sparkly flares on with a cropped, denim pink top, which sucked my boobs in and left my stomach drooping out for the world to see. I desperately accepted a wide, glitter-shedding-with-every-move black hat to cover my identity best.

'Perfect Meg. You look banging!' Lyssa exclaimed, admiring her creational efforts. I nodded back with a wry smile, and moments later, we were heading out the door and into a taxi. I almost knocked the hat off on the door, but thankfully, Lyssa had tied the string tight to my chin, so I went everywhere with the hat.

Prizm soon appeared into view. A building as tall as it was wide, one of Cardiff's biggest nightclubs. Lyssa had the taxi abruptly stop in the middle of Saturday night traffic, directly opposite the expanding queue to get in. Lyssa clambered out of the taxi and dragged me behind her. She started twisting her hips and laughing in the direction of a tall boy wearing an open white shirt who gave her a suggestive look. Meanwhile, I felt so self-conscious I barely looked up from the ground.

'Meg? At a club? Didn't think it was your scene?' A voice from behind said quietly. I felt a weight thump me hard in the centre of my chest.

'Are you alright, Meg?' Lyssa said, waving an arm in front of my face.

'Yeah! Sorry!' I said, refocusing my brain on her. I didn't see anyone else looking at me; that was weird.

We were knee-deep in the queue now, surrounded by people in their best outfits, ready to have a great time. The girl behind us was wearing a bright green mini skirt with an even smaller tank top of the matching colour. Her face was saturated with shiny, bronze makeup, and she wore thick, black eyelashes so long they would reach the club before she did. Looking over at her friends, she saw that they were all wearing identical outfits, but each was a different colour. One was orange, and the others in bright yellow and hot pink. A packet of four classic highlighters sprung to mind. I admired their confidence for a moment, and my eyes took me to the group of boys they were waving at. Five boys, all around the same height, got to have been six foot something, were hyping each other up.

'Go on, Jamie lad!' One of the boys slapped this Jamie across the back with his dustbin lid-sized hands, to which the guy shunted forward a bit from the force. His sandy hair shook as he laughed.

'Leave it out,' another boy with slick back black hair wrestled the other off of Jamie. Before I knew it, they were all piling amongst each other, laughing and winding each other up about which highlighter they fancied the most. I'm pretty sure the hot pink one came out on top. And fair play, she wore it very well.

Before I knew it, we had our ID checked and were granted access to the club. A bouncer welcomed us into the entrance lounge, and the lights were so low that I could barely make out the people from the tables and chairs. People were everywhere. Literally, everywhere. Some guy had one arm on the wall and the other in his pocket as he was chatting to this girl who had her back against the wall. A group of girls looked like they were having a serious discussion right next to them, and others kept weaving in between them all. The acidic smell of alcohol mixed with body spray was firmly in the air.

'It's so busy!' I said to Lyssa.

'Haha, you wait until you literally can't move without touching at least four strangers at the same time!' Lyssa shook with excitement. Although that weight had landed back on my chest, looking at Lyssa, I saw that she truly loved this, and it was wonderful to see. I remembered I was there to spend time with her, which allowed me to relax slightly, although loosely speaking.

Time went on, and we had been to most rooms in the club by now. Lyssa had danced more in three hours than I had ever done in my lifetime. She claimed it was the boys that kept her fit. Meanwhile, I supported Lyssa from the side. I found it best to sit on the sofa that lined the back walls, as I knew no one was behind me and could keep an eye on her. I'd lost track of how many drinks we had between us. All I knew for sure was that after a few rum and cokes, I felt dizzy and sick, so I stuck to rum and coke without the rum for the rest of the night. No one could tell the difference by looks, at least. Although Lyssa took a swig from time to time and consistently told me, I should sue them for making my drink taste like dog shit. Seems you really can't kid a kidder.

'Come on, Megggggg!' She shouted from the smoke-lined dance floor. I reluctantly picked myself up off the sofa and headed towards her. My dancing was a joke. It was more like an awkward shuffle. I was also worried that my boobs were going to pop out of my top at any given second, hence the additional caution I gave to each stiff movement.

'Aghhhhh!' I turned immediately to the source of the scream. It was Lyssa. She clutched her nose with her hand, the other shaking so badly that her drink spilt in every direction.

'What's the matter?' I said worriedly. 'Are you okay?' She didn't answer me. 'Lyssa!' I tried to shout over the booming music. I put both hands on her shoulders, trying to get a look at her nose. Upon moving closer to her, I felt a hard object reject my foot from taking another step. I looked down to see a brick. A *brick*. I quickly put two and two together, picked up the brick, shoved it under one arm, grabbed Lyssa with the other and told her we were getting out of there. I guided her through the endless crowd until we finally got to the entrance of the club. I tried to ask one of the bouncers for help, but he had been radioed something moments before and had disappeared into the sea of people.

'I'm alright now, Meg,' Lyssa said with a snuffled tone.

'You've been hit by a brick and you're bleeding, Lyssa,' I said sternly. 'You're not okay!' I implored. Her nose, swollen up like a bloody pulp, eventually slowed itself down. I was so done by this point it wasn't even up for discussion. Lyssa, however, her clubbing longevity was not to be challenged. Even if it was a brick to the face.

'Nah come on, to dance floor for a few more songs then we go?' Lyssa said taking my arm.

'Lyssa, you can't be serious,' I said, stunned. 'It's not even funny!' I said, unimpressed, as she laughed. 'I'm literally going to sit on the side, watch, then catch you when you pass out either from drink or bleeding!' Lyssa simply rolled her eyes and took off to the dance floor. People naturally stared when she took to the floor, dancing slowly with her pale pink dress stained with blood. I managed to get myself a seat sandwiched between two girls who were far too drunk to notice me. Aside from no personal space, strangers and consistent noise it was perfect.

After sitting and watching people dance, fall, and dance a bit more, I noticed a tall boy in a Hawaiian top and balancing neon glasses on the bridge of his nose push a little stand through the crowd. It was stuffed with sweets and snacks. Skittles, Doritos, anything that made you salivate after drinking alcohol, he had it. Now, this was the best thing I'd seen all night. What I'd have given for a pack of sweets at that moment was quite concerning. He clearly saw me gawping at his stand and meandered his way through the crowd over to me. He'd surely have made a killing tonight. Work smarter, not harder, and all of that.

'I see you looking my way,' the boy said carefully as he arrived. Looking left and right underneath his shades.

'Well, it's the best thing I've seen all night!' I beamed, although he didn't reciprocate my excitement.

'So it's a one-time offer,' he looked shifty. 'No repeats, no strings, no names, no contracts and certainly no contact,' he listed as if rehearsed. He thought I was going to harass him? No offence to him, but he certainly wasn't my type. In fact, I saw him eyeing up another boy earlier, so I'm certain I wasn't his either.

'I'm just after the fruit pastels, nothing else, don't worry!' I smiled up at him. With that, he bent down out of sight and started rustling behind the stand. I looked to my left, and the girl who had blacked out only a few minutes ago was now staring at me, judgment swimming in her eyes. I guess food still wasn't cool for clubbing. With that lingering in my mind, I looked up, and the boy was still behind the stand. What was he up to? I wasn't going to worry about it at this point. Then, Lyssa appeared with shock splashed across her swollen and still bloody face.

'OMG, Meg. As if!' She exclaimed, followed by hysterics. 'I never knew you were into this kind of thing! Good for you!' The shock was audible. When I turned my head back to the stand, the boy had reappeared with two rolls of fruit pastels in his hands.

'Thirty quid then, please,' he offered me the tubes.

'Say again?' I asked worriedly. Did I just hear thirty quid? Hold on. My brain was flooded with all sorts of thoughts. A shocked Lyssa, a shifty boy...

'They're poppers, Meg,' Lyssa could see the cogs in my brain turn before I did.

'...What flavour?' I asked embarrassingly oblivious. The silence told me more than my conscious brain ever could have.

'...Drugs?' I said slowly. *Drugs.*

'I'll be off then!' The boy took the hint and quickly ran his trolley away from us. I almost bought drugs. Oh my God! I put both of my hands over my head. Drugs. No wonder I had some looks. If it wasn't for the expense, I would have bought them too! So, after a brick to the head and an almost illegal exchange of the recreational kind, we finally caught a taxi home, and while Lyssa entered a stage of nocturnal bliss, I stared at the ceiling reflecting. I vowed never to go clubbing again; I'll never know why I thought clubs, and I were a good idea in the first place. I flicked my watch over and saw five am, I was tired, stressed, had a headache, and I couldn't help thinking how I could have done with was a real fruit pastel after all of that...

Need.
Sleep.

CHAPTER
Twenty-Six

COVID-19

Thankfully, I had no more run-ins with dodgy sweets at clubs, only essays and presentations as uni took hold of us in the new year. I worked hard but made sure to come down from it, too. Usually, Bea and I would find something to do together, whether at the cinema or out for a meal or a walk. It was like I'd known her for most of my life, and it worked perfectly to motivate each other to stay on the course. However, come March 2020, like most of us, our uni experience was cut short as the Coronavirus pandemic hit the world. The headlines were terrifying as what was thought to be the most unpredictable virus for a long time had struck our population. So many people were deemed vulnerable to the threat of the virus; those who were deemed elderly, immunocompromised, asthmatic, among many more. They either faced debilitating consequences of contracting the virus or equally fear of it. We soon realised the true danger of Covid as it claimed lives and left thousands critically ill. Consequently, uni closed and sent all of their students home. Those with practical aspects of their courses, like midwives, nurses and paramedics, for example, years two and three, were still to attend placement. However, the first years had been cancelled entirely as we were deemed 'non-essential', apparently in the most respectful way. I was glad to be deemed a non-essential worker and thankfully returned home to my family as the only silver lining I could take from it. But if I could have traded the pandemic for uni, there would be no contest. Covid took a close friend of mine and, unfortunately, like many others, left many of us lonelier than ever.

Come April, there was barely any good news anymore; Covid-19 was quite literally everywhere. I remember being allowed one walk a day for half an hour, to remain at least two metres away from anyone at any given time, and a trip to the supermarket became the highlight of our week. Thankfully, my grandparents were all independent and stayed shielded in their respective houses. My parent's household was healthy, so for us, it wasn't anywhere near as traumatising as it was for others. Horror stories flooded the news and social media. So many people's lives have been snatched or detrimentally altered as a result of this vicious disease. Whether it was adverse effects on your health, crumbling businesses leaving people financially compromised, or redundancies, we all suffered to some degree. I remember feeling so depressed that I turned my phone off for five days at one point and truly lived in isolation.

As for maternity services, the system was upturned. One study estimated that Covid may have contributed to around fourteen percent of maternal deaths between 2020 and 2022, but most researchers admitted it was hard to pin down exact causes with so much happening all at once. However, research for Covid often came with its limitations. For the best part, professionals could only estimate that Covid -19 may have contributed to deaths rather than being a direct cause due to a multitude of different factors. Regardless, it provided an exceptionally scary time for all. Due to its unpredictable nature, so many precautions were actions, e.g in terms of any midwifery appointments, only the pregnant person was permitted to attend. Alone. The same was true for hospital admissions, including birth. If there was ever an emphasis on the need for midwives to be able to build trusting rapport, it was during the pandemic. Partners, family members, and friends couldn't be there for the labour of their loved one or be there when their baby enters the world. A truly unbelievable time that undoubtedly left many with a suboptimal experience to say the very least.

Uni continued online and for us, which was the least of our problems. It was missing out on critical hospital-based placement in March, April, June and July that we had to worry about for the long term. The NMC only reduced the number of hours needed to qualify. That was all well and good for being on track to finish the degree on time, but with four months less of placement, we would have to work a lot harder to be up to standard. How would I get around 200 proficiencies signed off in year two? By the time Covid hit, I'd only had community placements, so all the hospital-based ones still loomed ahead. On the positive, I claimed a refund on the uni hall rent as we wouldn't be returning, sunbathed in the back garden with the dog, who clearly thought lockdown was the best thing ever. I passed year one, which wasn't so bad. But again, I had the only positive effect of the national lockdown. I'd never been as grateful to have been deemed low-risk and healthy.

Eventually, a vaccine was developed during the later months of the year, and many people classified as vulnerable were inoculated to slow the spread, mitigate the effects and ultimately save lives. Covid bubbles came into effect in the summer, when we could visit another household but only meet outside and had to remain two metres apart. The thought of seeing loved ones for the first time in months was blissful; however, when it's your seventy-eight-year-old Grandma standing with a visor on, it chipped away at my happiness, knowing how vulnerable she was and how deadly this virus really was. I'd have given anything to hug her; it was almost a year until I hugged her again, and I've held on a little longer every time, ever since.

Thankfully, when year two came around, vaccines were in play, restrictions were much less, and life was slowly normalising. We just had to pray it wasn't going to resurface out of control, although we all knew it would and certainly did.

YEAR 2

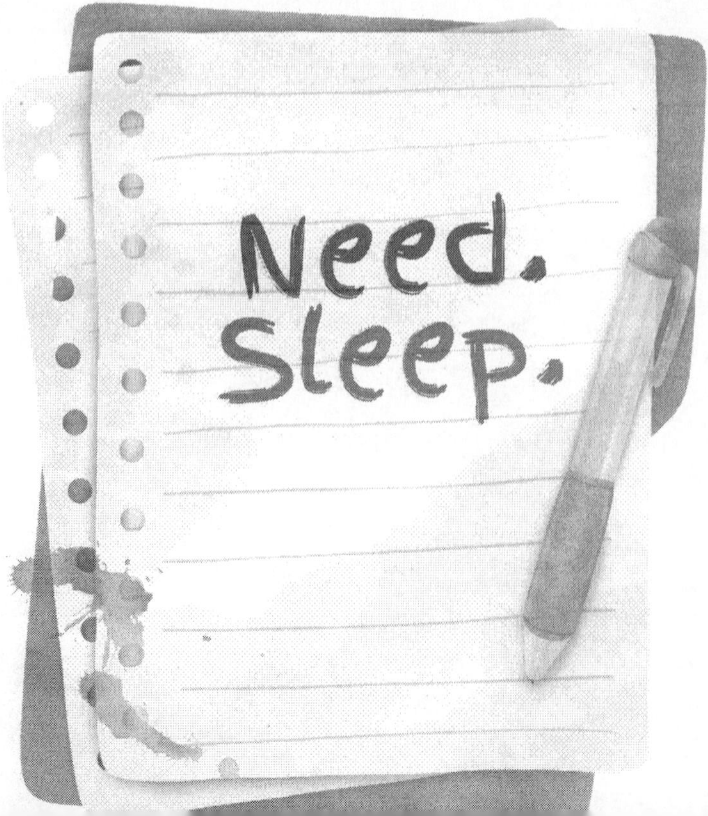
Need.
Sleep.

CHAPTER
Twenty-Seven

PAINTING, PERINEUMS AND PROPOSALS

I reached over my desk to the doorknob to let my sister in, who was rapping at my bedroom door. I stretched over my desk to reach the door, just as she decided to bash her way in anyway.

'Bollocks!' I hissed as my elbow smacked a glass of paint-brushes, sending murky water cascading over my freshly finished painting, a distorted witch holding a pumpkin that seemed to grow the longer I stared at it.

'What is that, Meg?' Al asked in disgust whilst standing in the doorway, eyes watching the paint run off the edges of the paper onto my desk and my lap. I pushed myself back from the desk and tried to avoid the mini stream.

'Well,' I stood there, stretching my trousers before me and shaking them. 'It was supposed to be a witch holding a pumpkin for Halloween,' I said glumly, looking down at the mess.

'Ohhh, I thought it was you holding a basketball,' she said, deadpan. Brilliant. I smiled and shoved her arm simultaneously, which sent her back an inch. I enjoyed painting rather than having a talent for it; I wanted to say 'I paint' to people when they ask what I like to do in my spare time.

Al turned my attention back to my laptop, which was whirring as if it was going to take off.

'Meg, are you supposed to be doing something?' Al asked her voice a mixture of curiosity and concern.

'Ah, yeah, it's perineal trauma today,' I said whilst stepping out of my wet trousers to get another pair on. Many lectures remained online to keep the spread of the still lethal Coronavirus to a minimum. I expected Al to carp at the 'filthiness' of midwifery training as she described it before, when yet another perineum was displayed on the screen, although nothing. I looked up in response to the unexpected silence and found her staring at my laptop screen instead.

'They're mentioning your name in the box,' Al said, scrutinising the screen. 'Someone called Estelle is asking for your opinion?' Al said informatively, scrolling through the messages tab. 'Are you the only Meg?' She turned her head over her shoulder. A) Estelle was the one running the lecture that day. B) I was indeed the only Meg. Abandoning my trousers, I hurled myself towards the laptop and felt my heart fall out of my arse hole. Eyes darting across the text, I found that Estelle had been asking for my diagnosis of the type of tear on the board for the last three minutes! With no reply, she'd started questioning if I was even there. In a state of panic, I quickly glanced at the poor woman's perineum on the screen. To be honest, there didn't seem to be much of her perineum left to inspect, so I assumed it was the worst, a fourth degree (for those lucky enough not to know, that's the worst kind, going from vagina to anus. Ouch) and pressed to turn on my microphone. However, my laptop did what it did best: buffered, the fan became louder, and the circle of doom appeared.

'NO!' I shouted whilst slamming a fist on the side of the keypad. Unaware that it had turned on my video, my whole body, from my stomach to my knees, was now showing on everyone's computer screen. There I was, unwillingly portraying myself to all of my fellow cohort. To the lecturers. To every other student midwife in my cohort. I felt my mouth go furry as I said the words 'fourth degree' hoarsely. Feeling as though my life had been drained out of my body, I dived to the left of my desk, onto my bed and out of sight. Mortified and unable to show my face, not even looking up to Al, I scuttled over to the side of my bed, stretched my arms over the desk (into the soggy painting), fumbled with the keyboard until I managed to click to turn the mic and video off.

After a few seconds of contemplating my entire existence, I peeled my forearms off the painting, transferring the remnants of a sloppy witch and an orange blur onto my skin. I covered my face behind them. Al was still on the other side of my desk behind my door, eyes wide open, covering her mouth so I couldn't see her laughing. Although, of course,

I knew her better than that. We both stayed frozen in the moment until we heard a voice emerge from the speakers.

'Meg, please don't worry or be embarrassed about this; technology often fails us; we appreciate you trying to fix it at the expense of yourself!' Estelle said sensitively. 'You also were absolutely correct with a fourth-degree tear; thank you for your effort to give me the answer!' Estelle exclaimed and went on to explain what a fourth degree meant. I switched off. I looked up in shock at Al, who now had tears streaming down her face. As far as I was concerned, I was experiencing fourth degree embarrassment, tearing from dignity to despair. Estelle at least assumed I was trying to fix my computer and not hurrying to change my clothes after a painting session that had gone everywhere but the paper now.

Hearing my phone buzzing, I picked it up, and it was going nuts. Al walked over and peered over my shoulder. Both of us were laughing at this point. I found lots of messages on the uni group chat. One from Brittney, 'OMFG Meg, you dirty devil'. Another from Vicky, 'What on earth have you been up to in this lecture, Meg? You should teach us a few things!!!'. That last one had a wink-faced emoji signing it off. Bollocks! They all thought I was doing something filthy. If they thought that, then what did Estelle think? Oh. My. God. I typed a message innocently explaining the disappointing reality, but the message of disbelief flooded in regardless. Realising I wasn't going to convince them and accepting the eternal embarrassment, I opened the chat between myself and Bea, who was also behind one of the computer screens. I frantically tapped the screen.

Me - 'BEA. BEAAA. Please tell me that didn't look as bad as it felt.'

She replied immediately.

Bea - 'Meg! What are you like? We saw it all!!!!'

Bea - 'And the panic dive onto your bed.'

Bea - 'I was wetting myself laughing. Classic Meg behaviour! Why were you even standing in your pants to start with? Xx'

I responded to every sentence and tried to justify my actions.

Bea - 'Of course you were. Did you not think to just type and say you were having Wi-Fi problems and couldn't turn your mic on or something? Kerrie did that earlier, and God knows what she was up to. I saw her story about 20 minutes ago, and she's not even at her house! Xx'

Why did I not just stop and think? I could be so literal and honest, or rather stupid sometimes. To think I could have saved all of the trouble with a simple sentence was slightly soul crushing.

Me - 'I just panicked and didn't think!'

Bea - 'Clearly Xx'

'Meg,' Al reclaimed my attention.

'Ahh Al, sorry I forgot you were even there then, no offence,' I said whilst swiping clear of the never-ending messages.

'What did you actually come in for? In a nice way?' I asked, remembering it was her who knocked.

'Well, the thing is,' she said slowly. I nodded. 'It's Slimy Sam,' she said plainly.

'Next door...' I said with caution, thinking this better not be another attempt to gain my hand in marriage. I was not in the mood.

'He's outside, in a suit, with a bunch of flowers, yet again asking why you said no to going out with him...and wondering if you'd be up for a socially distanced date in his garden?' She was low-key smirking. I slammed both hands on my bed in annoyance, he developed a crush on me during the last however many years, which fortunately for all of us involved, wasn't reciprocated by me. He would be wonderful for someone, I'm sure, but not me. Clearly, he hadn't got the message, so I made my way to my window to look out at the garden next door, which was filled with towering nettle bushes and a trampoline that was so rusted that it looked more like an extension of the ground itself. There was no path anymore either because the weeds had claimed it over as their own. Covid may have stopped many things, hence the plea for a socially distanced garden chat, but it only stopped human-to-human contact, not human-to-lawn mower contact.

Lost in the new world that was Slimy Sam's garden, my eyes wandered to two faded beige deck chairs that were virtually touching each other as they were positioned on the sole clear spot of the entire garden. Al read my mind and tapped me on the shoulder.

'Those were our spare chairs, remember?' She prompted me. I realised as soon as she said it.

'They were white, Al,' I said dryly. With that thought lingering, I flung my door open and bolted to my brother's room at the front of the house.

'Oi Meg, you need to actually wait after you knock, not just knock as you come in,' His voice boomed. Joe was thirteen and upon entry, he was sitting on his bed flicking through his phone. After sensing the urgency, he left matters to us and resumed his phone scrolling as Al, and I hurled across his room to the window. I opened it and shouted.

'Sam!' A splodge of a boy looked up, and a wide smile grew on his wide face. He was, in fact, wearing a suit. A dusty brown suit with sleeves too long and trousers too short. A part of me felt sorry for him.

'I was wunderin if you wanted to have a chat in the garden later?' He asked hopefully. I sighed. He hadn't got the message.

'Sam, I've told you before, I am not interested! I'm sorry, but my answer hasn't changed in two years and today isn't any different!' I exclaimed, but he continued to stare longingly at me. 'No matter how many flowers you bring to the house, how many times you send me messages through the letterbox, I'm sorry, but the answer remains the same,' I said firmly. 'We're just not suited!' I added just for clarity as this had got to have been the twentieth time I'd told him no. He'd been asking since I was seventeen. I'd only hoped he would get bored and move on.

'So you did get my notes then!' He said astonished. 'But you never replied to em,' he hung his head sadly. I felt a pang of guilt but most of it was annoyance it had to be said.

'Marsh deals with all mail and filters out the crap; you'd be better off asking him!' I added a little angrily now. Al and Joe both laughed behind Joe's blackout curtains with visions of a Marsh taking the post and burying it under the big green chair, which he often did, it wasn't a lie.

'So, do you want to then or not?' He persisted. The memory of a fish, I swear.

'NO!' I slammed the window, ran back to my room, told Al I'd see her later and sunk to the floor, still in my viral pants looking at the state of my room and feeling the state of my witch. Dishevelled. I noticed my laptop had run out of charge also. At least there wasn't anyone other than myself in my room now and I didn't have to share my reflection with thirty others.

I started to worry about what had happened, but the worry slowly turned to amusement. What on earth! Why was it always me? After twenty minutes or so of clearing up the mess, plugging my laptop in, sending an apology email to Estelle, and slowly getting the order back to my life, I flipped my phone over and found another message. This time from Mum. 'Al just told me! You nutter. At least you're all midwives there, could have been worse!' I smiled down at her response. 'I've also sent Sam packing! He knocked on the front door not so long ago; something about Marsh being part of Royal Mail? What on earth did you say to him? He'll be bringing his parcels to us next!' I laughed, dropped my phone, danced to Wham, and welcomed chaos like an old friend as we hurtled, hand in hand, into year two.

CHAPTER
Twenty-Eight

A NEW CHAPTER

After what felt like 700 years of online lectures, we were finally allowed to move back to uni in late September. We'd levelled up: no more crumbling halls, we were proper adults now (sort of). Five of us became six, including Bea this time. We had bagged a beautiful house right opposite the uni gates.

A) An actual house. How I'd missed it.

B) Intact shower nozzles that actually worked.

C) A commute so short I could practically roll there. Life was looking up.

Mum and Dad came and helped me move everything back to Worcester where we got to work Megfying my new room. This time, no breakdowns over walls or plumbing.

Growth. With Disney scattered across my new space and some newfound calm scattered across my heart, I said bye to Mum and Dad as they made their way back to Wales. Al had GCSE meetings the next morning and Joe needed to be dragged to school; he was following in my footsteps with his own miserable school experience. Kids could be dicks, I should know. With my parents safely back in Wales, I could settle into the new normal. And what better way to embrace normality than with a bit of ridiculous chaos? Bea and I got back to adventuring wherever possible.

The 'How Am I Still Alive?' Tour: A 2021 Highlight Reel:

- Inflatable assault course on a lake? Brilliant idea. Until I slipped on bird shit, flew off the platform, and resurfaced to find poo between my toes. Nearly vommed.
- Online lecture? Cosy. Bea and I cocooned ourselves in Sherpa blankets... until Lynsey outed us halfway through. Warm? Yes. Subtle? No.
- I started talking to a boy through a friend of a friend. Seemed normal. Then he told me he liked listening to me breathe. I sleep like Darth Vader. Of course I attract the unhinged. I blocked the guy so hard, he couldn't even find me on twitter.
- Bea fell between two hotel beds thinking they were connected. I laughed until I cried. Cheers, Bea, finally chaos I didn't cause.

- Found out I was returning to X. The rage made me accept a milkshake laced with Jack Daniel's. Left the restaurant horizontal. Another never event.

Chaos was great, but it couldn't distract me forever. Reality was calling, and it was wearing scrubs.

First placement - Delivery Suite. My stomach churned at the thought, I was a second year with zero experience. Don't get me wrong, I was excited to get stuck in, but my subconscious was freaking out. It was the big unknown, like being told you were heading into space and had to navigate it without NASA. What also cranked up the pressure was the sudden upgrade in midwifery theory. The lectures were so much more confusing than year one's, as we'd now launched into the world of complications, building on the so-called 'fundamentals.' We often blamed Covid for everything, clinical gaps, social awkwardness, our general confusion, and honestly, we weren't wrong. I only hoped the trust had been forewarned to help us out more and judge a little less. Again. So naive. Still, if midwifery, and life, had taught me anything, it was this: nothing ever goes to plan, but you show up anyway. Helmet on. Scrubs ready.

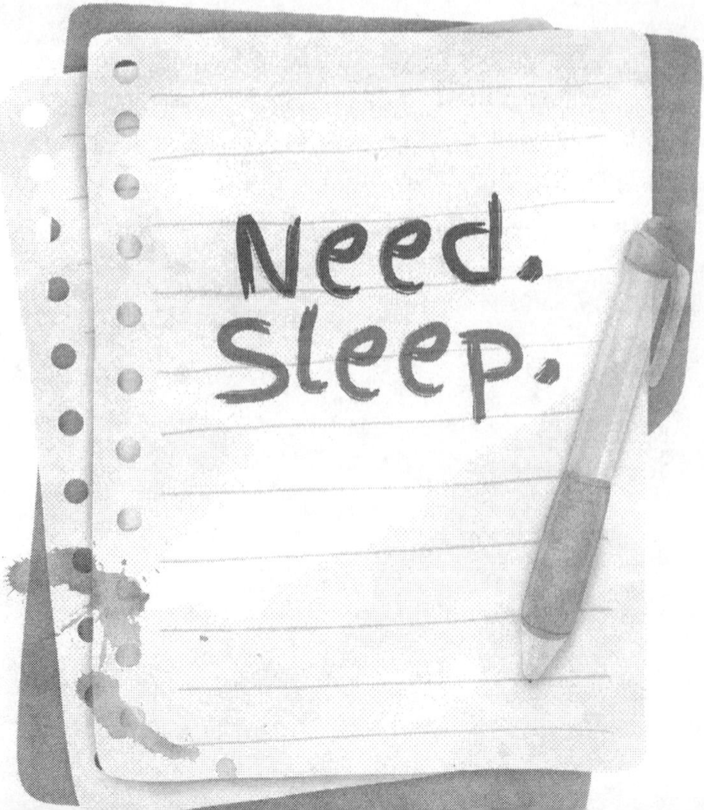
Need.
Sleep.

CHAPTER
Twenty-Nine

SARGENT SANDRA

The brain is brilliant at building psychological defences, tiny internal alarms triggered by past pain. One bad encounter can make you wary of anyone who even vaguely resembles the source. Midwifery training turbocharged this reflex. Between Letitia's contempt and the relentless pressure of unpaid full-time work, my mental shields went up fast. But nothing reprogrammed my brain faster than Sandra, my first mentor of second year.

ACT I: STUDENT AUCTION

I RETURNED TO THE TIRED-LOOKING COUNTY HOSPITAL on a crispy night in October. What had once been a quiet hospital before the pandemic now felt utterly barren. I made my way to the second floor, through the bare corridors and onto Delivery Suite. In every occupied room, thin violet-coloured curtains were drawn across the open doors, protecting some of the dignity of the patients they harboured behind them. I took a deep breath of anticipation and let a sigh of stress straight back out. Whether it was returning to placement after a year, the pressure or the isolation of Covid-19, probably all three, I asked myself if this was really for me. Not having long to question my life choices five minutes prior to the shift handover, I heard a midwife say that Doreen wasn't in today. Who, typically, was the name of the midwife I was allocated to work with. I felt panic creeping up on me as the midwives each took a turn to scope me out. They darted their eyes from my face to my name badge to my uniform and even my knees at some point. What did they have against my knees? My mind asked my body desperately to leave, but my body seemed to be unplugged and firmly stood stationary until it was ushered by another member of staff to 'stop blocking the doorway'.

Unblocking the doorway, I fell into the changing room, where I realised it was like a broom cupboard. Tiny. I reviewed the faces of those I'd be working alongside for the night; one had hair that extended to her backside, and her face did the same. Another put her blues on and looked like a supermodel, but was she really living the dream? And the third gave me a wry smile, to which I nervously introduced myself.

'I'm Meg, great to meet you,' I said shyly, to which she returned a small smile. Before I knew it, I followed the blue bodies back into the corridor and into another small office for handover.

The supermodel turned out to be more of a super midwife (the shift lead), and I watched as she took handover from the other midwife in charge, who looked as though she hadn't eaten or even breathed for the last twelve and a half hours. Little did I know, this was a rather accurate presumption. Following the confusing handover of all sorts of words, terms and names I either hadn't heard of yet or knew very little about, the allocations began.

'Who are you working with?' The supermodel directed her question towards me.

'Was supposed to be Doreen, but I don't think she's in?' I replied with doubt despite knowing it was correct.

'Okay, any takers?' She opened the floor of the auction for me. However, no one offered a bid or even looked over the ad to consider what was on sale. I looked around the room to find the long-faced midwife looking down at her legs, another one in scrubs scratching her head, and eventually, everyone was looking the other way, not wanting to take 'the student' as the supermodel had labelled me. So, she allocated me to a midwife called Sandra.

'Brilliant, thank you,' I said gratefully. Sandra, a short, blonde-haired woman, shot her head in line with mine and squinted her beady brown eyes tightly in scrutiny. Before I had the chance to think of a way to deal with the uncomfortable eye contact, she raised a hand to her brow and threw a salute, yes, a salute, out into my line of view.

'Year?' Her voice was short and sharp, like her features.

'Beginning of second,' I responded quickly and somehow brightly. I got a stare that could have turned the most robust of stomachs. I could see her mind judging every part of me. Was she assessing my ability based only on appearance? If so, she was bound to classify me as incapable, seeing as my face was practically painted with a portrait of uncertainty.

ACT II: SANDRA'S QUIZ FROM HELL

Once we were finally out of handover, I recognised a recently qualified midwife who I knew as a third-year last year, exiting room five and heading towards us. We took handover, and I had never felt so lost. Terms and abbreviations flew around my ears, none of which going in. I had no idea their meaning or even what they were related to. Mum? Baby? Me? The dog? No idea. I remember just praying she didn't quiz me, as my vacant expression would only worsen.

Clearly, there wasn't a God to help me in my time of need, and just as if my thoughts had teleported into her mind, she raised her hand to stop Kate from speaking. Looking on edge herself, Kate turned to face me as Sandra was. The first question of tonight's game show was asked in front of Kate and the rest of the midwifery team as they were all sitting at the same desk. She hated me. Already. It was going to be one long night.

'What is a PCR test, and how would you interpret the results?' She asked blankly. PC what? Plum? From Balamory? Trying to dissociate the idea of PC Plum turning up on his bicycle in a minute to rescue me from the PCR test, I tried to think of any possible answer to give her. 'Pulse' had to be in there somewhere, right? Sadly, my ability to focus was torn by her continuous stare.

'Umm, I'm not too sure, sorry,' I managed to find a response, as crap as it was.

'Right, well, I'm not telling you; you can research it for yourself,' she said with a nasty twang. I felt a ping of anger dash along the side of my body. I'd be caring for a woman I had no idea what was going on with, look incompetent, and face eternal embarrassment. This was a literal nightmare.

'Question two: Why do we give magnesium sulphate to PET ladies?' She asked robotically. I'd never felt so stupid; I had no idea. Again, we hadn't covered the depths of that yet.

'Sorry, Sandra, I'm not sure of that either,' I said sadly. She rolled her eyes so much that I lost her pupils to the back of her head, and they weren't coming back anytime soon. To be honest, I was surprised they didn't fall out of her skull and head for the exit, as I wanted to do so desperately do myself...

'And why don't you know this either?' She shot at me. I looked to Kate, who smiled at me passively; pity weaved through her eyebrows. This made me feel like I needed to cry for eternity.

'We just haven't been taught it yet; we haven't really completed first-year hours yet,' I tried to defend myself weakly through a voice break. I found my eyes glistening with a film of emotion and had no other choice but to look up. I slowly glanced from the ceiling towards my fob watch, which was resting on my bigger boob of the two, Jupiter. Unfortunately, my left breast is a little smaller and has Saturn status; it was a natural choice as the second-largest planet in the solar system. Trying to forget about how well my breasts can impersonate the solar system, I noticed eight o'clock on my fob; my shift didn't end for twelve whole hours yet. Holy shit.

The horribly long handover quiz showdown finally ended, and Kate sadly left us, making me feel more alone than ever. It was just Sandra and me for the evening, night and early morning. What was I actually going to do?

'Where are the drugs room and things, Sandra?' I asked to distract her.

'Follow me,' her command style was less Nightingale, more Napoleon. She got up with quite some speed and began to march. She genuinely strode with her arms as straight as a board, swinging alternately by her side through the ward's corridor. I noticed her perfectly pinned ponytail didn't even move the whole time. Even her ponytail was uptight. How was that even possible? I frantically tried to keep up with the speedy march through Delivery Suite. Owing to the fact that I carried a proportion of the solar system on my chest, I weighed probably two of her. Maybe even three. Therefore, I found it even harder to keep up with her, especially in tight-fitting trousers and what felt like a straight jacket as it held my upper arms captive. She flew past the front desk so fast the others didn't look up; Sandra was on a mission. Unfortunately, when I staggered past the desk, they all looked up in sync, as I was practically jogging after her at this point. Their response was to snigger over the sound of rapid inhalation fading as quickly as it appeared as I disappeared after my leader. Suddenly, she came to an abrupt stop and swivelled around as though presenting The Weakest Link,

'I haven't got time for this. Do you know what a fire extinguisher looks like, or do I need to ask you to research that, too?' She spat at me. I hung my head low. I had been reduced to not even being able to recognise a fire extinguisher. A red canister labelled 'fire extinguisher'. Clearly, I was living in the prime of my life. I just stood there in silence and waited for the next blow.

'Fill in the gaps tonight. Or return to first year,' she said plainly. 'Oi,' she shouted loudly. Thinking it was for me, I looked up instinctively. However, I could only see the back of her ponytail. She was summoning a fellow student. God bless her. I looked up and sent a prayer to the sky. The girl immediately removed herself from the main desk and hurried towards the corner where we were standing. As she got closer, I could see she was slightly built, with her familiar glossy hair swirled neatly on the top of her head in a bun. You couldn't mistake that, it was Gracie. My heart breathed a sigh of relief. She was not only a friendly face but an ally; she was from the same cohort as me, so she knew how awful our unique situation was.

'Hey Meg, you alright?' She said softly to me, to which I nodded whilst fighting back tears.

'Could you give this student a tour, please? I believe it's her first day in the unit,' Sandra asked Gracie in a much nicer tone. 'Oh, and don't rush returning her to me,' she went on to ruin that nicer tone. Gracie and I exchanged a look of 'you're safe with me for the next thirty seconds', and it was exactly what I needed at that moment in time.

ACT III: PRINTER HUDDLE WITH GRACIE

We walked very slowly to the end of the corridor and out to the main intersection, where we dipped into a corner behind the printer. I hadn't seen that level of hide and seek since I was in year eight when some worrisome students were trying to waste time before returning to maths from the 'toilet'. However, I understood exactly why they did this now, as when Gracie and I crouched down, I could have let it all out there and then. We whipped our paper-thin masks off our faces and simply exhaled. I knew I was safe to speak.

'Gracie, I can't even tell how good it is to see your face, who are you with tonight?' I asked with a fair share of concern and curiosity.

'Mate,' she raised her hand to rest on my shoulder. 'It's great to see you too but having to deal with Sandra on your first day, that's shitty,' she said, screwing her face in disgust. Understatement. I shook my head in response. Gracie laughed and repositioned herself to signal she was settling in and had no intention of returning. I found myself doing the same. Both of us are resting our backs against the wall now, me with my feet pressing against the printer and her knees bent up to her chin. She rested her head on her knees, and I could see the understanding in her eyes.

'It's actually shit here, isn't it,' she declared honestly.

'I'm actually starting to hate it. I just feel useless, and what's worse, the midwives know it, too,' I replied solemnly.

'Me too, babe, don't sweat it; they just enjoy making you feel like shit. Makes them feel better about themselves,' she fairly spoke. 'Don't worry though, I literally came in the other day, and Lisa, do you know Lisa?' She awaited my recognition.

'Blonde and tall?' I tried to put a face with the name.

'Nah mate, short,' she shook her head. 'Either way they can be knobs, and we shouldn't have to put up with it,' she told me with some sass. That's what I always admired about Gracie; she knew her self-worth.

'Paha, stop it. I'm not even sure If I can make it past nine o'clock at this rate!' I laughed for the first time in what felt like forever. Although it was sad to hear, I was reassured that it wasn't just me going through the shit. Maybe it was a student thing? But then, according to the trusty sources of other friends' experiences in other trusts, there were some horrible people everywhere in life, but the negative encounters didn't seem to be this frequent. We found mentors hit brilliantly, or you missed terribly with no in-between.

'Do you know what PET stands for?' I asked desperately.

'No?' She replied blankly, 'let me try and google it,' she tapped quickly on her phone. Was I about to be thrown a lifeline? 'Sorry mate, no signal,' she sighed. The universe had not thrown me a lifeline after all.

'Ugh, I just don't see the need for making us feel small,' I said, knocking my head back onto the wall after a while of reflection. 'We're here to learn and all; otherwise, we'd be midwives, wouldn't we?' I found myself saying with a touch of fury. This was the aspect of training that frustrated me the most over the three years. If every student knew what they were doing, they'd be a midwife, not a student midwife. Time for a call for more supportive staff for the student body; maybe the NHS would retain a few more newly qualified midwives. They wonder why the dropout rate is so high at almost sixty per cent of student midwives leaving.

ACT IV: HUMILIATION ROUND TWO

After slating the midwives and warning each other about names to avoid at all costs, we finally decided to return to avoid suspicion. Sandra was back at the computer, and Gracie's mentor had just made tea in the staff room. I reluctantly peeled myself away from Gracie and sat awkwardly in the chair next to Sandra's, staring blankly at my handover sheet, pretending not to read the same three words over and over again: PET. PCR. Magnesium Sulphate. My brain whirred like a computer trying to open a file that wasn't compatible with its hard drive. PET lady, someone had said earlier. What did that mean, was she a gerbil? Had midwifery extended its scope to the rodent population? I couldn't even Google it. No signal. No Wi-Fi. Just yesterday's dog photos and my food diary waiting in the void, completely useless. I moved on to magnesium sulphate. I knew, or at least I thought I knew, that magnesium sulphate was given to pregnant people to offer their baby neuroprotection should it be born too early or to mitigate severe pre-eclampsia symptoms and even seizures (all very true). The keyword, though. Pregnant. Why couldn't it be PE lady for pre-eclampsia? It would make much more sense. What was the T?* Even so, the problem with this was this 'PET' lady, was that she had her baby in the cot at her side. So, unless she was planning on a refund by means of sticking the kid back up there in the attempt to cook it for a little longer, what use was Mag Sulph now? To be honest, I could have done with some myself at this point, maybe it would have given me some neuroprotection and further brain development, as clearly, I needed it*.

'Can you take manual blood pressure? It's important,' Sandra stared directly into my eyes. After some deep thought and longer than I want to admit, it clicked. PET: Pre-Eclampsia Toxaemia. *Toxaemia*. A serious hypertensive condition in pregnancy. Of course. We'd only brushed past it during a rushed online lecture in lockdown, probably while I was still trying to work out whether I'd accidentally muted myself on Zoom. My brain had been spinning like a dial-up connection trying to load that file. Not a gerbil. Not a dog. A very unwell pregnant woman. The 'T' didn't stand for Terrier - it stood for the terrifying consequences if not treated properly.

'PET is Pre Eclampsia!' I said happily confirming my suspicions.

'Yes. Pre Eclampsia Toxaemia in its full term, PET,' she said plainly. Why couldn't she have said this from the start rather than deliberately keeping it from me?

'So, can you? Take a manual blood pressure?' She repeated.

'Yes!' I replied brightly. Thankfully, I bought one on eBay for twenty quid during lockdown, and it quickly became the best purchase I had ever made.

'Right, well, that's good as your second-year knowledge,' she paused to shrug, 'is getting quite embarrassing, really, don't you agree?' She went on to ask. I felt those words being etched into my brain right at the front of my introspections of placement, which had remained for the best part of my midwifery training. I unintentionally held on to how she made me feel so small influenced my lack of confidence for a long time.

'We've only had twelve weeks of community placement to date,' I said nervously. 'We had a whistle-stop tour on a load of emergencies etc., and at the end of theory block, which was all online, we were told to swap our stripes and learn on the job, so, I'm sorry that makes me rubbish at this moment in time,' my lips began to alter shape as my chin wobbled. Thank God for face masks, the dreadful pandemic had given me something after all. A place to hide my emotions whilst I was strengthening my backbone. I thought I saw a flicker of surprise in her face. To this date, I always wondered what she was thinking at that moment. Was she pleased she made me angry? Was she doing it to toughen me up? Was she cruel to be kind? Or was she just cruel to be cruel?

A few hours passed, and Sandra commanded me to follow suit. At two-thirty, she silently dragged me over to the ward to go and get 'methyldopo' or something. Was it a dance? A Greek cheese? A new indie band with the next number one?

'Methyldopo, Sandra?' I asked. I understood how annoying I must have been, but I had to ask as I'd never learn otherwise.

'You don't know what methyldopa is for?' She looked at me with disgust. 'You're telling me you went through the whole of the first year not knowing what methyldopa is for? Are you joking?' No, Sandra, the last thing I felt like doing was cracking jokes with you.

'No,' I answered flatly, regretting my brutal honesty technique. She stormed ahead, and I followed sheepishly.

We arrived at the main desk of the Maternity Ward to find another midwife sitting on the desk, the desk bending slightly under the pressure of her weight rather than the printer she moved to sit there. Sandra asked how her shift was going. So maybe she is capable of basic people skills. The midwife replied with the usual.

'Stressed, so fuckin' busy!'

'Guess what, this one doesn't even know what methyldopa is for! Can you believe it?' Sandra turned to me with amusement splashed across her face.

'Well, you'd better get Googling that one, Sandra's not going to be happy with you,' she laughed. Brilliant.

Back on Delivery Suite, we refocused our attention on our PET lady, not in the gerbil sense, as it was time to give the magnesium sulphate alongside the standard anti-hypertensive medications (usually, labetalol or nifedipine or methyldopa, sometimes a bit of them all), which didn't seem to be doing a good job at stabilising our patients' blood pressure. The risk of it running too high is problematic for the body as a whole system, but the threat of a seizure or stroke is quite simply one of the biggest and dangerous threats for obvious reasons.

'This will be good to practice how it's drawn up; at least I've learnt a lot tonight,' I said optimistically.

'Oh no, no, no. I don't think so!' She almost laughed. 'You don't even know what it is; that's an error waiting to happen,' she snapped. 'You can stand in the corner and watch me.' What a joke. I slump off to the corner of the room with my hands cupped in each other, resting in front of me. I felt like a child sentenced to half an hour on the naughty step. I tried to peer to see some action, at least, but I couldn't. Every time she caught a glimpse of me moving, she'd pause, and I'd get the hint and bow my head in shame.

The shift didn't get much better from there, although Sandra said less and less to me as the night advanced which was a positive for my tolerance levels at least. And so, with Mag Sulph in hand and a confidence rating of minus seven, I trudged into the rest of the shift wondering whether I should google 'how to become a florist' when I got home. Florists don't need to know what methyldopa is for.

And so, eventually, after what felt like an eternity, that truly painful shift ended. Inevitably, feeling empty yet so glum, I rolled up at the drive, and after making sure I'd parked my car safely, I remember I bashed my head down onto the steering wheel and cried for a while. When most of my body's water content had left me, and I felt slightly more together to get to my room without detection, I went into the house. I entered and instantly saw Amy getting up for work. Bollocks!

'Ahh, Meggie,' she said kindly. I tried to contain myself. 'How was your shift?' She enquired. *Shit, I'm never going back.* I answered in my mind.

'Alright, thanks! Knackered now, though, going straight to hit the hay! See you later!' I said in one breath and disappeared quicker than Sandra's military march down the corridor of Delivery Suite. I entered my room, sat on the floor and sobbed.

I was so knackered that morning that I cried myself to sleep and didn't wake up until about four p.m. I stretched, peeled myself out of bed, and headed downstairs for a cup of tea.

'How was last night?' Harriet was behind the open cupboard door this time and gave me a good scare.

'Was alright, thanks,' I said as neutrally as possible.

'That didn't sound convincing,' she provoked a further response. As if she pressed a button inside of me, I felt my eyebrows fold and I evicted my pent up stress through my tear ducts. Ugh. Crying into my tea bags, my life began to fall apart for the fiftieth time over Sandra and the hundredth time in my degree (I wasn't even at the halfway point). I ended up telling Harriet everything, and she was horrified.

'What the fuck Meg, that's awful!' She wrapped her arms around me until I felt uncomfortable. Later, I ended up spilling it to all of the girls who encouraged me to go through the speaking up algorithm, as they called it in uni, aiming to educate practice supervisors about any discrepancies amongst students and staff. Deep down, I knew it was a waste of time as she was an experienced staff member and was well respected. But I agreed to think about it at least and we had a day of self care to recover. We all went out for a meal and put the world to rights and later Bea, and I went to a dance fit class (I almost died, but at least it was very effective at refocusing my mind).

So, the human brain sure does create powerful protective mechanisms when it has experienced danger and thus acts in defence. My brain added Sandra to the mental rolodex. One more trigger. One more shield. I wasn't sure if it was making me smarter, or just harder to reach. Regarding this particular person, I'd found out from a trusty source some months later that, amongst other errors, the said midwife had been fired due to giving the wrong dose of something to a woman in her care. I enquired to trusted staff members about where she'd gone. Apparently, there have been numerous complaints about her practice, attitude, and overall safety. Unfortunately, it looked like I wasn't the only one to have had a poor outcome from the Sergeant.

*Toxaemia. Pre-Eclampsia Toxaemia (PET). Sadly not a small rodent in a bonnet.

*It was only later on that I truly understood the use and power of magnesium sulphate for a wide range of reasons; neuroprotection for prematurity, inhibiting pre-term labour and birth, mitigating symptoms of pre-eclampsia potentially preventing the deterioration to eclampsia and seizures and so much more (which I kind of knew). What I was confused about at the time was its equally important use in both the antenatal and postnatal women. People with PET can certainly havre seizures postnatally, therefore, trusty magnesium comes into play.

CHAPTER *Thirty*

THE HOKEY-COKEY

A few shifts after The Sergeant, I was beginning to rebuild my confidence, which, admittedly, was powered by a potent blend of panic and determination. I spent most of my free time researching anything and everything so they couldn't humiliate me again. But I was starting to realise that theory only got you so far. It was practical midwifery that taught you what you really needed to know.

This time on Delivery Suite, I was with a midwife who actually explained things and let me ask questions without acting like I'd just pissed on her shoes. It was... refreshing. So, Leah and I were looking after a woman whose labour had a slow start but eventually shot her baby's head out like a cannonball*. Unfortunately, she had a particularly nasty tear that needed suturing. One of the doctors came to do the repair but was called away to an emergency just before the end. They asked Leah to give the diclofenac suppository, something midwives do anyway. Fine. No problemo. Just a simple task of popping a tablet up someone's bum. When we explained what it was and how it worked, the woman and her partner got the giggles. Fair enough. But they laughed so hard that the tablet fell straight back out. Leah said she'd never known that to happen. So, she popped it back in, only for it to ping out again like a little pharmaceutical yo-yo. Every time the woman laughed, out came the diclofenac. Eventually, Leah cracked a smile when I muttered, 'When I picked up a leaflet about midwifery, I never imagined I'd be doing the Hokey-Cokey with anal drugs at five a.m. on a Saturday morning.'

When we finally managed to keep the tablet firmly in situ, we slumped down with a cup of tea to write the notes. Leah turned to me with a deadpan expression and said,

'I've got to the last bit. About the diclofenac. How do we even start with that?' She dropped her head into her hands and started laughing.

'Put your diclo in,' I said, trying to keep a straight face. 'The diclo fell out, in out, in out, shake it all about...'

'We do the Hokey-Cokey, and she pops it back out, that's what it's all about!' Leah finished the song off, and we completely lost it. That magical five a.m. delirium worked wonders for bonding.'Cheers to PR dic,' she added, then immediately realised what she'd just said. Another eruption of laughter.

So truly, thank you, per rectum diclofenac. You've been good to me.

*As I'd learnt from baby Enid back in 2019, the more controlled the head delivery, the better for minimising perineal trauma. Some of the smoothest births I've seen - thanks to a combo of manual perineal protection from us midwives and Olympic-level panting from mum - still ended up with spectacular tears anyway. Sometimes it's just the way the anatomy crumbles. But as a general rule, if you want to keep your vagina more or less intact: pant, don't push, when it feels like your entire lower half is on fire and a melon's making a bid for freedom.

*Diclofenac - basically long-lasting ibuprofen, but in suppository form. It's delivered via the back passage (per rectum or PR), and very effective, especially considering it's being administered right next to the injury site. Efficient and humbling.

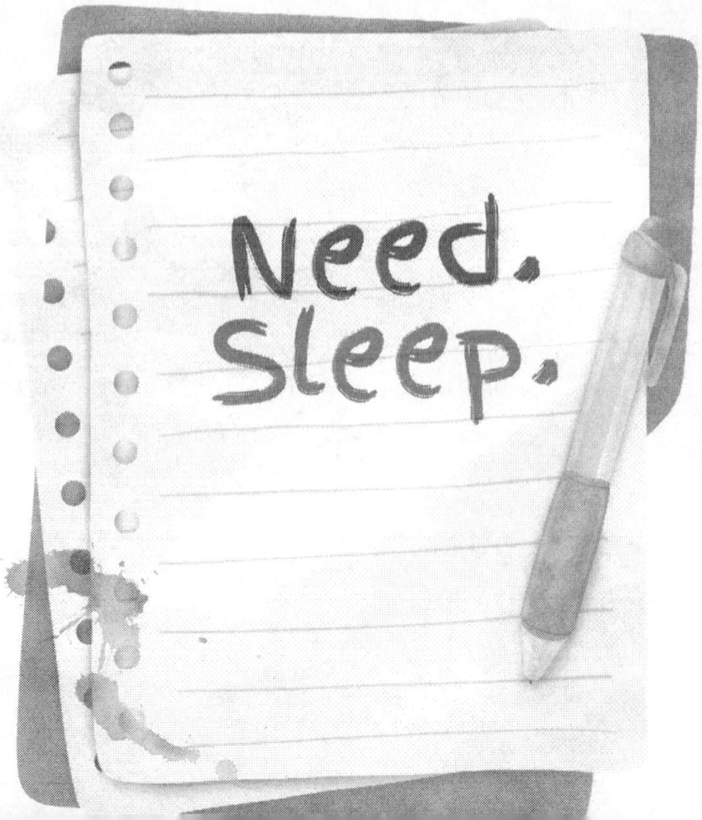
Need.
Sleep.

CHAPTER *Thirty-One*

DEVASTATION

PART ONE — THE BIRTH

As my training progressed, I began to understand why midwives rank so high for burnout. Don't get me wrong, there are incredible moments, absolutely. Birth can be euphoric, powerful, uplifting. But the highs are high, and the lows...well, the lows can crush you. I learnt that the hard way, during one shift on Delivery Suite with a midwife called Vivienne. Vivienne used to be in senior management, but when I asked, she said she'd stepped down to do a few clinical years before her retirement. She said being back on the front line meant everything. I admired how she had devoted her life to midwifery, which was something I couldn't envision for myself at that stage, I felt the pressure way too high to be sustainable. Maybe I'd feel the same one day, who knows?

Anyway, we were given a woman, first baby, thirty-nine weeks who was seven centimetres at three thirty, therefore, plan for reassessment as we came onto shift. Vivienne helped me have the confidence to try a vaginal examination, it was my first labouring cervical examination, and it was the strangest thing. Once my fingers reached far enough, they were blocked by a hard, spherical head. When I swept my fingers across the head to feel where the cervix was in relation to it, I realised I was feeling the baby's hair which was a strange sensation as they were very much still unborn. I felt like a contestant on I'm a celeb, where you have to blindly put your hands into a hole and find the star. I always thought I'd like to give it a go to see if I could handle it (I probably couldn't), so who knew I was sort of living it in my own way? Anyway, there was only a small amount of cervix left that I could feel so I forewarned the woman it may be wrong but guessed her to be nine centimetres. Vivienne rechecked and confirmed that she was between nine centimetres and fully dilated, with a small piece of cervix left; some thing I've come to know as an anterior lip. The plan was to give two more hours before offering a repeat examination to see if that lip had gone and we had reached full dilation. No cervix left meant the transition into second stage of labour; all things birth.

I busied around, mostly following Vivienne, as admittedly, I knew my experience was limited still. So, I orientated myself to room three (I'd not been in there until this point), started to get familiar to where the pads were kept, new sheets and gloves. Although, when our patient asked for a sick bowl quickly, I opened the drawer full of needles instead. Helpful. After my initial embarrassment, it turned out sick bowls would be the last thing to worry about as when I next auscultated the fetal heart rate, at about 08.15, I heard a slow thump...thump. I turned immediately to Vivienne who was hacking away at the keyboard.

'Doesn't sound like a decel*, probably maternal pulse, don't worry,' she said casually. I remember feeling stupid and tried a different place to listen, but the next contraction happened rapidly, and the woman told me to get off of her. So, I left it and after a few moments, I listened again, to find that same sound. I palpated mums heart rate too and her's felt quicker than this. I remember feeling like my own heart was going to drop out of my arse when I turned back to Vivienne.

'Vivienne, this is definitely different this time,' I tried to be as calm as possible. Vivienne came over, took the doppler and had a go herself which was what I wanted her to do the last time. She felt the woman's abdomen and tried a different place where she got the rapid drum of the FHR which was a relief until what she said to me next.

'See? Maternal pulse,' she implored. I blamed myself for probably scaring this family for absolutely no reason, even though something about what I heard felt different. Did Vivienne just brush me off? Or was I simply clueless and still had a long way to go? This time, I genuinely had no idea.

Not half an hour later, that same dulcet beat filled the room again. Vivienne suggested a repeat vaginal examination in case the baby was imminent, and Libby agreed. At five past nine, Vivienne confirmed baby's heart rate had settled back to normal and that Libby was fully dilated. She advised Libby to follow her urge to push. However, the baby wasn't about to arrive in the next few minutes. It's perfectly normal for first-time mums especially to spend up to two hours in the pushing stage, and how well the baby copes can influence whether any intervention becomes necessary.

Libby pushed with the urge, and each time she did, we saw movement of her external anatomy - a reassuring sign that she was pushing effectively and in the right place. During second stage, fetal heart auscultations are performed more frequently, every five minutes. The first few were normal, which was a huge relief. But by nine thirty-five, there was still no sign of the baby, and that scarily low heartbeat returned.

'Do we need a CTG* now?' I asked Vivienne nervously. I didn't have a good feeling about it. The baby clearly wasn't going to be born any time soon, and by now I was sure I'd heard a few decelerations - intermittent, yes, but without a CTG I had no real sense of the bigger picture. Or was that the problem? Maybe I was relying too heavily on machinery to tell me what was normal or not. Maybe I just didn't know enough yet to trust my own assessment. I knew that was part of being a student - but the uncertainty still felt dangerous.

'No, don't make the low-risk high-risk, Megan,' she replied with certainty. 'Right, I'm going to sort a few things, so any problems, Megan, shout me,' she encouraged me and left the room. I felt the most uneasy feeling flood my veins.

'Do you think he's okay?' Libby asked me directly as soon as Vivienne had left. I wasn't prepared for the question - or maybe my face had already betrayed me.

'I'm sure he'll be okay, yes?' her partner, Andrew, said quickly, pulling her into his arms. They both looked at me then, waiting for reassurance I wasn't trained or experienced enough to give. What was I meant to say? In healthcare, you can't promise anyone anything really. All you can do is assess what's happening in the moment and act accordingly to try and optimise health and prevent adverse outcomes. It is the art of juggling health, safety, and the sheer hope that nothing decides to go pathological before you've had your morning tea.

'Do we need to go on the monitor?' Libby asked, her voice thinner now. She meant a CTG. She wanted certainty, and I didn't have it.

'It's better for me to speak with Vivienne quickly before I put you on it,' I said, trying for confident but hearing the wobble in my own voice. Libby and Andrew exchanged a look, the kind of look that said 'we've lost trust' and my stomach just dropped. Vivienne was nowhere to be seen, and the tension in the room was rising like steam. The uncertainty felt too risky, too heavy to ignore. When Libby asked me again, I pulled open the drawers, found the straps, and started a CTG at Libby's request, hoping it would offer the reassurance none of us could.

The CTG wasn't too bad to begin with. Baby's baseline was behaving itself, with the usual second-stage variable decelerations - good old head compression doing its thing. But there's a thin line between "totally fine" and "please someone call a grown-up," and I was still learning how to tell the difference. How much do you back your knowledge when your knowledge is basically still on a trial run?

'Why have you started this?' Vivienne asked as she re-entered the room, and I felt like I was going to evaporate.

'Mum's request,' I said quickly to which she pursed her lips together.

Five minutes later, the baby's heart rate had dipped to seventy beats per minute and stayed there for three minutes and counting. That was enough to prompt Vivienne to hit the emergency bell, and an entire army of staff came charging into the room. Well... "army" turned out to be two midwives. The unit was tiny on the best of days, and everyone else was already tied up in their own birthing rooms. One midwife announced that the doctors were dealing with an acute emergency in theatre, and our senior midwife was wrestling something urgent in triage. Brilliant. What on earth do you do then? Pray? Manifest? Bribe gravity?

'Onto your left side please, Libby,' Vivienne said, and together we helped her roll into the left-lateral position - the one that takes pressure off the vena cava and hopefully boosts oxygen to the baby. Thankfully, the fetal heart rate crawled back to normal after the position change. Relief, but the kind that still leaves your stomach in your shoes. We needed an obstetric review... but without an obstetrician, that was going to be tricky.

Vivienne slipped out of the room again, this time saying she was going to return with the registrar. I wanted to believe her. I really did.

'Can we still have a vaginal birth if baby's distressed?' Andrew asked as he put both of his hands on the back of his head.

'We might not have time for that, it really depends on what the doctor thinks of what is safest for you and your baby to endure, I'm sorry I can't be more sure for you both, I'm very much still learning about it myself,' I said honestly. With that, Vivienne re-entered, the woman was like a yo-yo. But she brought our in-charge midwife, where was the bloody registrar?

'This is, Bethanie, our senior midwife, our doctor is still with another emergency in theatre but will come as soon as they are finished.' It's almost like she heard my internal, preceding question. Bethanie introduced herself, agreed that baby needed to be born soon, as the CTG was showing further concerning characteristics now.

So, whichever way was quickest and safest, both parents were on board. Thankfully, Libby pushed very effectively in the doctor's absence and push after push, baby's head was visible. Vivienne and I coached Libby to push as hard as she could to see more descent and hopefully birth, however, baby barely moved. Bethanie prepared the equipment needed for an episiotomy*.

Three to four minutes of another sustained deceleration, and it continued without recovery. No one pulled the emergency bell this time. Was it because our most senior person available was already present? At five minutes, there was still no birth. At six minutes, Vivienne performed an episiotomy to expedite delivery. There was no immediate effect. By seven minutes, the fetal heart rate remained significantly depressed, and I felt completely frozen. Thirty seconds into the seventh minute, the baby was delivered by sheer maternal effort.

He was extremely pale, with poor tone and no respiratory effort. Was this presentation consistent with severe perinatal compromise or an immediate and physiological response to a bradycardia? Vivienne immediately clamped and cut the cord to avoid delay and transferred him to the resuscitaire for neonatal resuscitation. I activated the emergency bell. Additional staff entered rapidly. I will never forget the atmosphere in that moment - a palpable, collective fear shared by everyone in the room.

I channeled all of myself onto mum and dad and did my best to support them and talk them through what was happening, but, in the absence of a cry, they were understandably impossible to console.

'Is he dead? Andrew he's dead, I know it,' Libby shouted hysterically as she tried to get a look at her little boy.

'His heart rate is okay, we're trying to help him breathe now,' Bethanie said from the resus.

'Oh god, Meg, what happens if he doesn't?' She turned back to me, a face full of panic.

'The team are doing everything they can for your baby, I can promise you that much,' I said sternly as she flung her arms around me, her terror pressing into my bones.

Baby was successfully resuscitated at ten minutes of life and the pure concoction of conflicting emotions in both Libby and Andrew's eyes over-spilled into a stream of relief and terror in equal measures. Baby went to neonatal unit for breathing support and eventually was transferred out to a tertiary unit for more extensive care. I remember sitting in deathly silence in my car at the end of the shift. I couldn't bring myself to drive for a long time. I had so many questions. I watched the trees repetitively sway in the breeze and wondered if this was what it was like to feel nothing. Similarly, when I eventually arrived back home, the jarring normality of my bedroom felt wrong after what I'd been a part of.

A few months later I received the news that I had been called as a witness for the events leading up to baby being born and the immediate postnatal period. It turned out baby had suffered a degree of brain damage and therefore, a Serious Case Review (SCR) had commenced. I remember the feeling of my heart sinking like a heavy stone to the pit of my stomach. My thoughts extended to Libby, Andrew and baby Edward if they stuck to the name they told me about at the time. I thought of them consciously and subconsciously, waking up at night and remembering baby Edward's face as he was born. Did we do something wrong? Did we not do enough? These questions went round in my head for months. The images replayed repeatedly, sometimes vividly enough that I'd consider staying awake just to avoid reliving them in my sleep. I still think about them, even now. I wonder how they are, what their lives look like, and whether everything turned out well for their son. I want to believe it did - that he has a life filled with stability, happiness, and peace. But the truth is that I will never know, and learning to live with that uncertainty is its own kind of weight.

PART TWO — THE FALLOUT

All in all, the process of the SCR was nothing short of terrifying. I remember being asked what happened between the clinical note I wrote at 08.40 and 08.50. Every action at every time was understandably under scrutiny from the perspectives of every professional personnel present. I tried to remember every detail and answered as accurately and detailed as I could. I felt it went well considering. However, once the interview had terminated and the recording had stopped, the interviewer thanked me for attending and showed me to the door. I distinctly remember her saying 'good luck with your training, you're clearly going to need it after what's happened.' It left me with a bit of an empty feeling in all honesty, something I couldn't quite put a name on. Was that code for I was to blame?

I headed slowly toward Delivery Suite; at least they were expecting me to start late. I got changed on autopilot, then set out to find my mentor, trying to shove my racing thoughts into every corner of my mind. It was the last place I wanted to be, especially after reliving the worst memory of the place moments before.

'Megan?' An unfamiliar voice asked.

'Um yep that's me,' I quickly flicked my eyes to her badge 'Rhian' and smiled, I'd not met her yet.

'How on earth you are sat on this seat when Vivienne's been forced out?' She hissed. Was she serious right now? 'Do you realise how much of an amazing midwife she was before you pitched up?' She asked with a nasty shadow darkening her features.

'I, um, she's gone? I had no idea,' I stuttered. I knew I was the last to be interviewed but surely, her leaving was long before this day, as I'd only just had the interview?

'You should be gone after what I've heard, putting a CTG on a low-risk woman without even asking the qualified midwife,' she stopped abruptly as another midwife entered the break room. I was hoping they would be my saving grace and this bitch, Rhian would be forced to terminate her horrible mission to beat me down.

'I was just saying about Viv, Bex,' she publicised the subject of conversation without hesitation. I could feel my face burning up and eyes prickling with increasing panic.

'I just need to go to, well, before I start,' I tripped over my words and then my own feet as I clambered out of that chair and into the corridor of Delivery Suite. My heart rate had soared, and it felt as if my heart was thrashing around in the cavity of my chest. I ran straight for the abandoned block of toilets on the ground floor of the hospital and cried until I didn't have anything left to give. I went around a million and one thoughts; what had I done? Had I caused a baby harm? Where was Vivienne and why had she gone? Was it a delay to put her on the CTG? Was it not escalating for help sooner? What if there was a doctor available? Would this be any different? Maybe it was my fault for not being braver and starting the CTG earlier. What have they heard? What have they said? Maybe I should leave after all.

I spent three hours on the toilet floor before ringing my mum and reliving it all again. Mum was furious, cried with me from time to time and told me to return home as soon as I was fit to drive. I went back to uni that day, switched off my phone and lay on my bedroom floor for the rest of the day and into the early hours of the morning. I eventually got into bed and stared at the ceiling for the remainder of that night. Each self degrading thought had etched into the core synapses of my brain.

- I'm not good enough.
- They think it's my fault.

- They hate me for it.
- What if it happens again?
- What if it really was my fault?

By the end of it, I'd talked myself into the idea that leaving might be the safest choice - for me, for everyone.

THE BREAKDOWN

Before this point, I'd never suffered with poor mental health, just the usual stresses that can be managed. I refused to believe I was struggling for a long while after this event, but that's human nature, denying is your defence... until that defiance becomes your detriment. Over the weeks I started to feel as though life was quite weirdly pointless and that we were putting ourselves through the fires of burning hell and back to simply die and become dust...a thought that was wildly unsettling and bleak. This mindset combined with horrific mentors making me feel like I was in fact already dead, done and dusted, pushed me over an edge I didn't think existed.

I spent the next few weeks on high alert; I'd flinch to anything and anyone and felt I couldn't trust the world and that it was quite an awful place. I spent my days off crying or having panic attacks about baby Edward, me as me, and the hospital I was forced to keep going back to day after day, with some of the most vicious and intentionally horrible people I have met in all of my time.

Since qualifying and mentoring students of my own, I have learnt a very important lesson about this event; it was not my fault. I was a student working under the registration of a qualified midwife. Students are not qualified and therefore, do not hold any legal responsibility. It is the responsibility of the mentor to guide, supervise and act appropriately.

Fast forward to qualifying (hard to believe at this point, right?); I remember Mum said to me to give it a week at a new place and if I didn't like it, it may have been the midwifery. However, to this day, most of the staff at the trust I work for now, are nothing but supportive, encouraging and empowering. As with lots of things in life, it's who you share things with that has the biggest effects. You could go through the most horrific events, but from experience, you can either bounce back and find peace in a new direction or be beaten down into a shadow of yourself. Human to human connection is the most powerful force. It can quite simply make or break you.

But I also I think of Libby, Andrew and baby Edward more than I ever expected. They changed the kind of midwife I became. They made me more vigilant, human, compassionate, and unforgiving of people that forget we're all still learning.

*Decel - Short for deceleration. Officially constitutes of a decrease in the baby's heart rate for fifteen beats less than its baseline for fifteen seconds or more. Classifying decelerations is another degree in itself; some are isolated, some repetitive, they could be variable, shallow or late too. Whether they occur with contractions or without is also very telling and dependent on their features and clinical situation, the same presenting decel could be normal for a woman about to push a baby out but abnormal for someone not in labour. It's a law of its own and one of many very good reasons for needing three years of training and annual updates for.

*CTG - Cardiotocograph - Two spherical monitors strapped to the abdomen; one transducer recording the FHR and the other, an ultrasound, recording pressure, i.e contractions. We also have a maternal pulse probe too for obvious reasons. The idea is that we are able to assess the baby's heart rate over a period of time giving a picture of how they are coping. However, circumstances are ever changing, and the most terrifying part is that if you have a normal CTG at 10.00 say and you take it off. When you next listen in at 10.15 say, the FHR could have stopped. A CTG shows what's happening in that moment of time and previously. Research and evidence continue to battle between whether CTGs actually have predictive value, however, the latter is that when we identify signs a baby is not coping, we can expedite birth and potentially save a baby's life. It's another complex thing.

*CTGs have different classifications based on their features. It's a little bit like a traffic light; reassuring/normal (green, to continue), non-reassuring/suspicious (amber, start to implement some conservative measures) and pathological/abnormal (in most cases whatever is going on needs to stop, i.e stop labour and for birth of the baby, quickest and safest way).

*Episiotomies are the art of making a controlled incision to the perineum to aid the birth of the baby in cases of fetal distress or to prevent more severe perineal injury. We infiltrate the perineum with lidocaine and then take the epi-scissors to the perineum, a couple of centimetres long. They sound dreadful, granted; however, they can be the difference between a good outcome and a poor one for mum, baby and sometimes even both.

CHAPTER
Thirty-Two

HAPPY FORTIETH

A bit of a 180 now for this next one. It's a story of laughter and light, which given the previous, is much needed. This is a true representation of midwifery, life in the NHS if ever there was one; you can have a day when the worst happens, and twelve hours later, the sun is shining on hope and happiness again. Sometimes, you've got to hit turbulence before you can cruise through the smooth. So given that I was feeling like my mind had caved in on itself, I decided to return to South Wales and spend some time at home with family before returning to my next shift. Mum and Dad absorbed my emotional overspill and helped me navigate the more stubborn emotional knots too. I still felt hopeless as I couldn't see past not passing the course and therefore, make nothing of my life. Although, following a wonderful mix of time with my nearest and dearest, commencing sessions with a counsellor and a plan from GP; they helped push me in the right direction and I was able to start seeing the sun through the clouds again. I felt a lot of heavy emotions still, and many days were still quite grey, but I was able to a laugh again, which I found was the best type of medication, and where this next story came at a good time.

I eventually returned to Delivery Suite and after a few shifts with positive midwives, I was progressing well. I was finally seeing my theoretical and practical knowledge overlap, gave me those 'holy shit, it makes sense' moments, and a little tickle of oxytocin as a reward. Don't get me wrong, there was still a steep hill ahead of me, but I'd started effectively shovelling some dirt at least.

My mentor for this account of events was kind but didn't say much, so we kind of balanced eachother out. We were looking after room four, where a couple navigated their way through the labour of their second baby. A Maroon 5 playlist softly rumbled from the computer speakers, and the lights were dimmed to be a low buzz in the background. Their baby moved a lot, which they said he did when Maroon 5 played. The kid had a good ear for music already. Marie was relatively comfortable, given she was four centimetres. Between contractions, she was busy chatting away with us, and the latest topic was how she and her wife Liz had both hired bouncy castles for both of their fortieth birthdays last year. I got really into the conversation and was chuffed to hear you could get away with being a big kid at any age. I remember discussing hiring a theme park and dreading how much that would cost in between documenting.

'What did you do for yours in the end, then, Meg?' Marie said as they both turned to await my response.

'Your fortieth?' Liz smiled as I didn't respond. *My fortieth.* Sorry? I was nineteen at the time, not even halfway to forty. I only left college a year ago and passed my driving test the year before that. My eyebrows lifted themselves a considerable distance upward from the sheer shock, and my face broke into a smile. They'd ask me for my fiftieth plans in a minute, and I'd be peeling my eyebrows off the ceiling!

'Oh, not quite forty?' Liz laughed as she read my undeniable reaction.

'Haha, yeah, not quite,' I was unsure of what to say next. Should I admit I'm a teenager and prepare for judgment? Or roll with it and own my new age? I'd even put a few puffs of makeup on that morning, too, seeing as I was on a dayshift. It wasn't even like they had the excuse of a night making it hard to see someone. It was broad daylight.

I decided to laugh it off in the end and it went down as a topic none of us revisited. A few hours later, I was in the staff room preparing to leave as my shift ended. Marie had progressed well and was seven centimetres on leaving. They thanked us both for making their experience full of fun and laughter so far. I'm glad they enjoyed aging their student midwife by two decades. I felt my phone buzz in my bag and reached down to grab it. I had my car keys and a water bottle in my hand, so I answered the phone and sandwiched it between my ear and my shoulder.

'Hey, Mum, how's it going?' I asked as I shimmied through the double doors.

'Meg! I'm good. I'm quickly checking in tonight as I need to pick Joe up from his friends!' Mum said happily. I could hear the dog pitter-pattering his nails on the floor as he trotted around the house in the background. 'How was your day?' Mum said with a nervous undertone.

'Welllll,' I elongated my words.

'Oh god, what now?' Mum anticipated any answer.

'I've apparently aged twenty-one years since I started year two,' I said plainly. 'A couple asked me what I did for my fortieth birthday today! Plus, I'm sure I've spotted my first grey hair!' I laughed until I had to take a deep breath.

'That's hilarious! You must have been tired today!' she laughed. 'And there's nothing wrong with being forty, I'll have you know,' she chuckled on the other side of the line.

'There is when you're still technically a teenager, Mum!' I said as I envisioned my twenties and thirties skipping past hand in hand, laughing as they left me ahead of my time.

'Teenagers are more tired; you're still developing, its fact,' Mum reassured me. 'You'll find your get up and go with your twenties and thirties,' she said with a soft smile.

'They've got up and gone, Mum!' I said, and we both laughed until our jaws hurt. What had my life come to?

CHAPTER *Thirty-Three*

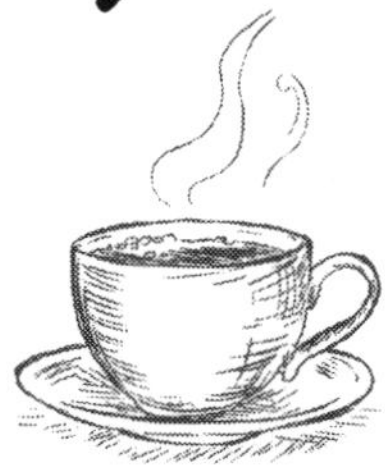

MEDICALLY UNFIT

Christmas was only seven weeks away, and my brain had never been so busy. The midwifery foundations of year one felt a different lifetime ago as year two included so much depth that the complications had complications. From additional care needs to obstetric emergencies, it was yet another world I had to attempt to comprehend. To add to the festivities of academic writing on critically appraising treatment for a complex condition, we also had to sit our second exam on medicine calculations. It was something we had to do each year to show we were concocting drugs on a safe level. The pass mark was one hundred per cent, as it is pretty simple: you are either a hundred percent right or hundred percent wrong when it comes to drugs. With no room for error, I had made a few posters to try and get it to sink in when I got up and dressed in the morning or came home from a shift, although mostly, I would face plant my bed and completely ignore everything else around me. At least the thought was there.

On another wintery day, I encircled myself in a blanket on my uni bed in the new house and looked at the surrounding houses. I kept thinking about how it was a massive upgrade on year one, a quaint estate and no green walls. I returned to the day's task, where I put in my AirPods and started the country music to see me through the upcoming mathematics. I found background songs that I knew inside out gave me the illusion of familiarity in unfamiliar territory. It made it manageable. It helped explain why I never particularly enjoyed silent school exams; I found the silence of the world around me only made my head louder. My type of brain always needed stimulation, always.

For example, even when watching a film or something, I needed to do something else, such as painting, drawing, or gaming. But a black-and-white exam paper with no sound around me just wasn't sensory focused for me. My brain overcompensated for the lack of things to focus on by causing distractions of pure havoc. Thinking back to that physics exam in year eleven, I kept repeatedly singing 'Yellow Submarine', by the Beatles instead of working out the dimensions of a prism. I didn't even like The Beatles. Or that time I was tapping my leg so fast and loudly in one of the religious studies exams that I was asked to step out of the hall for a few minutes. I ended up running in circles like a spinning top for a minute before I went back in. To be fair, I managed to finish the paper after that. In geography, I'd finished the paper with thirty-five minutes to spare. By the end, I'd played Snog, Marry, Avoid with half the six form. Still with time to spare, I'd invented a full romantic drama between the invigilators and decided that the man collecting papers was named John, an ex-hitman hiding in plain sight after framing his colleague Eileen for a murder he definitely committed. GCSEs? More like BBC drama pilot. Anyway, noticing pins and needles in my right foot as I had been sitting on it for so long, I tuned myself back to the country music and pressed 'start' on the assessment.

'Meg!' Bea was shaking me like a malfunctioning vending machine. I blinked. Was I dreaming? Nope. I was in my uni bed, draped in a blanket burrito and surrounded by the wreckage of revision.

'You had time to sleep, in a mock exam?' Bea asked stunned.

'I what?' I asked confused.

'You're unbelievable,' she said, plucking my AirPods out like she was disarming a bomb. 'You're smart, but that's taking the mic,' she said laughing. I wiggled the mouse of my laptop, and its screen flashed 'timeout' and underneath it '5% completion'. I dropped my mouth open in shock so much that I would need to pick my jaw up off the floor if I wanted it back.

'Remind me not to listen to country when I'm studying,' she said quietly. The country relaxed me so much that I fell asleep and missed the mock exam completely. It turned out mine was the last but one with the lowest ranking in the cohort. Bollocks.

'Who on earth got lower than you did, Meg?' Bea said laughing, as we all knew what happened with mine.

'They'd have to be dead or really stupid,' I laughed in return. The uni chat pinged off at that moment, and the person with the lowest score was Kelly.

'Don't worry guys, no one could've done worse than me x.'

She hadn't even started the exam. Her daughter had an epileptic fit and needed an ambulance. That's why she got 0%. I… fell asleep to country music. Suddenly, my joke answer about needing to be dead or stupid didn't feel so funny. 'Well,' I said, eyes wide, 'guess who's the stupid one.'

Bea snorted. 'Meg, this could only happen to you.'

CHAPTER Thirty-Four

A DIFFERENT KIND OF CONFETTI CANNON

I re-took the medication exam after I explained that it was my computer that had crashed, not my body's wake cycle. Annie believed me, and funnily enough, I passed when I answered the questions. With one more crisis averted, I turned my attention to my birthday, a January affair, which, let's be honest, is the calendar equivalent of trying to party in a grey Tupperware box. My parents always made our birthdays spectacular, no matter the time of year, but let's face it, January birthdays suck. Everyone's broke, hungover, or in a post-Christmas coma, so any provisional plans made in December vanish with the tree. Anyway, year after year, I always viewed it as a great excuse to blast out the January blues with a trip somewhere and cake. Always cake.

Considering my friends were unavailable for whatever reason, Bea and I had booked the Celtic Manor for a night. It was literally fifteen minutes away from my parents' house, but it was a grand hotel that sat on the top of a hill overlooking a neighbouring town, including our hometown. Just the two of us, away from midwifery for a while, with the idea to read a book, have a swim, and eat some good food. Perfect.

'Meg, did you see that Harriet is pregnant and is leaving?' Bea turned to me as I was driving.

'What! Not Harriet, really?' I sat further upright, both hands on the wheel. I'd flicked my eyes from my mirrors so many times they probably had one eye assigned to them by now that I was so stressed about being road safe.

'Shit, sorry, I forgot we were in the car for a moment; I was just so shocked,' Bea apologised for breaking one of our unwritten rules, which was not to tell me anything shocking whilst I was driving because because I couldn't multitask. Any dramatic revelation mid-drive usually resulted in a swerve, a drift, or a narrowly avoided hedge.

'It's okay. I am focused on the road,' I said comfortably as we turned off onto one of the A roads now. I noticed Bea's body language relax as we left the motorway and my seventy-mile-an-hour era behind.

'How did that even happen?' I resumed the shock.

'Do I have to draw you a picture?' She laughed.

'Obviously not.' I rolled my eyes. 'I mean, when did she have the time? I don't even have time to wee, let alone-' Then I saw it. A pigeon in the road, dithering like it couldn't decide between death and glory.

'Oh shi-' THUMP. Feathers. Everywhere.

'Jesus Christ!' I shouted as we drove through the plumage.

'Bloody hell,' Bea whispered, staring at the smudge on my windscreen like it was a murder scene. My eyes glossed over as I realised that I'd killed a bird, no matter how unavoidable it was.

'Don't ask me to draw you a picture of that one!' She tried to make me feel better.

We continued driving with only the engine doing the talking as we were still in shock.

'Wrong exit, Meg, first exit!'

'What?' I said as I came back into the present.

'We've gone the entire wrong way,' she groaned. I blinked. I couldn't concentrate after a pigeon explosion. My hands were still shaking, and now I had to U-turn past the carnage?

'You do realise we are going to have to go past it again now,' she said.

'Great. A second viewing. Maybe this time the ghost of the pigeon will flip me off.' Moments later, we had backed onto ourselves and were driving down the same road as a few moments ago. As we approached the scene of the incident, the road was covered in red feathers. I felt sick as we passed it, but I felt even worse when I saw another pigeon standing on the roadside, flicking its head side to side, confused about the remains of its mate.

'How did that even happen?' I asked Bea, as I'd never seen a pigeon literally shit itself to death.

'My mum says pigeons burst when they're hit because they're full of gas'. She described it like they are feathery little pressure cookers. I shuddered internally.

‘Careful, I might do the same after that trauma. Pop and everything,’ I shivered. ’Ahh, Bea, I feel so bad,’ I said sadly.

‘I know, it’s awful, Meg, but you couldn’t have done anything about it; he literally flew at you, plus you couldn’t swerve, etc., because you may have crashed and hurt us or someone else,’ she reassured me.

‘I thought it was pheasants that were suicidal, but pigeons don’t half make an exit.’ This was the January blues in full force: no one showed up to my birthday, and a pigeon exploded in my honour. Happy January to all.

CHAPTER
Thirty-Five

FAKE BLOOD, REAL FRIENDS

Despite the pigeon (RIP), Bea and I had a fairly uneventful stay at the Celtic Manor and found it helped us unwind, ready to face the rest of January. However, the peace was short-lived when February rolled around, and academic chaos returned with a vengeance.

On one particular clinical skills day at uni, we were let loose on the plastic arms to practice venepuncture and cannulation. Just a singular arm, from the shoulder down, sat on the table like a forgotten horror prop. Welcome to healthcare degrees.

'Alex, can you pump for me, please?' Andi, one of our lecturers, asked as she prepared to demonstrate venepuncture. One of our fellow students Alex clambered up beside the arm and grabbed the two hand pumps, which were attached to containers of red liquid and, of course, the arm. Alex pumped away while Andi palpated for a vein full of knockoff blood. She removed the cap from her needle and, instead of the textbook thirty-degree angle you'd use on an actual person, she stabbed in at nearly ninety degrees, because the plastic was so dense you'd need a jackhammer otherwise. Still, the fake blood surged into the tube like the real deal.

'Off you go!' she beamed, casually sticking a plaster over the plastic arm, as if that was going to help now. Bea and I were paired with Josie and Lottie, who we'd grown closer to since year two started. Josie was twenty-eight and one of the kindest, most grounded people I'd ever met. Lottie, twenty-five, had the same easygoing energy and an infectious laugh that could carry across the campus.

'Here we go,' Lottie said, cracking her knuckles like she was about to enter a boxing ring. Josie took the pumps, and Bea and I offered moral support as Lotte inserted the cannula tip, drew back, and.. 'I have a flashback! I actually have a flashback!' Lottie cried, spotting the tell-tale backflow of blood in the chamber. We all clapped and cheered as she advanced the cannula, withdrew the needle, and secured it like a pro. Josie and I followed suit, blood and all, success all around. Then it was Bea's turn, and I hopped up to man the pumps. Bea got the needle in, drew blood, and all seemed to be going well... until the blood bottle shot clean off the cannula. A fountain of red liquid sprayed out, coating Bea, Josie, Lottie, and the floor. Between the severed plastic arm, the blood-soaked humans, and the growing puddle of gore, the scene looked less like midwifery training and more like an outtake from CSI.

'Oh my god, I'm so sorry!' I gasped, staring at my best friend, who looked like she'd just been attacked by a rogue ketchup bottle.

'It's okay, Meg,' Bea grinned. 'Means I get to skip a bit of this and go home to change.' We all cracked up, even as fake blood continued dripping off the table. I decided I should at least try to clean up the chaos I'd caused. As I leant over the table to mop up the blood slick, my foot caught a hidden puddle underneath and, WHAM. I slipped and landed hard on my arse. The impact sent a new splash of red liquid into the air, which rained down on Josie and Lottie this time too. The room fell silent. I turned to see the rest of our cohort frozen at their pristine stations, wide-eyed and horrified. My face turned the exact colour of the floor. Bea looked like she might combust from laughter. I couldn't even be mad. Still, from that moment on, the four of us were glued together by blood. Literally. And metaphorically. Because nothing says lifelong friendship like mutual trauma, a fake murder scene, and a bruised arse. Silver linings, guys. Silver linings.

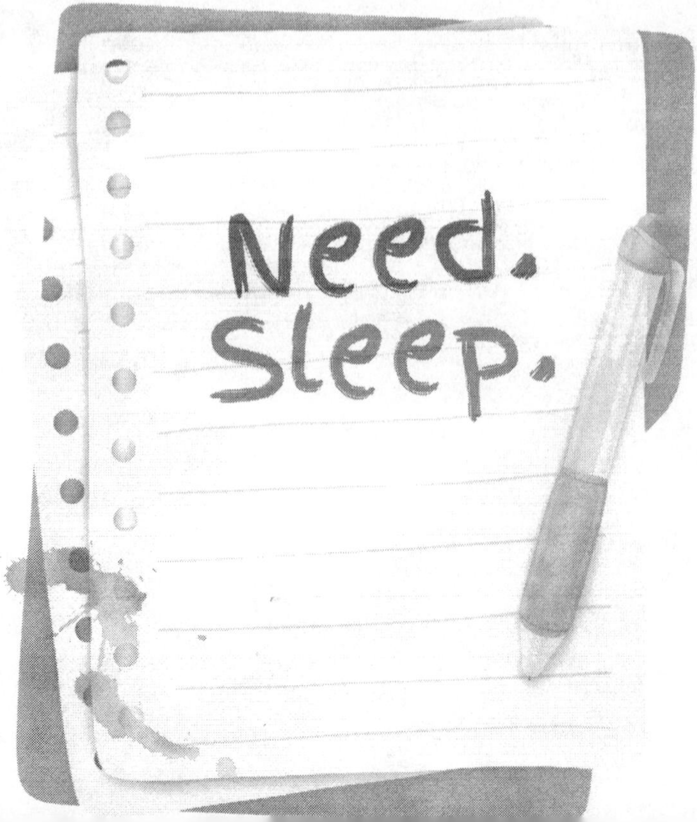
Need.
Sleep.

CHAPTER *Thirty-Six*

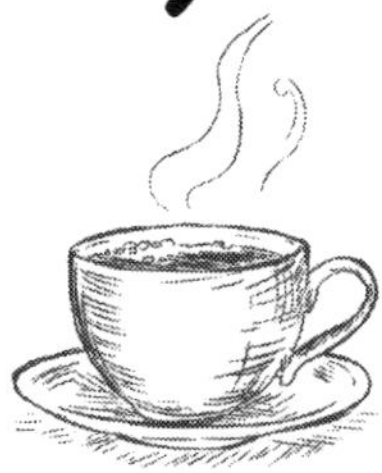

SIMPLY IRRELEVANT

I'll admit, theory blocks were a welcome break from twelve and a half hour shifts that left you feeling half-deceased. But what they saved in physical exhaustion, they made up for by melting your brain instead. If brains responded to overuse, like muscles do, I'd have been walking around with a neurological six-pack. Unfortunately, all mine did was hoard lemon muffin crumbs and stress. My body, neglected and sedentary, had given up entirely. Hours hunched over my desk, rereading the same academic article for the fifth time because it used words like 'epistemological framework' and 'paradigmatic lens,' left me one brain cell away from institutionalisation. The worst offender? Learning to 'research like a true scholar.' Apparently, that involved critiquing every source of research like a bitter coffee shop customer furious about how their drink was destroyed in every aspect. Research became my biggest bugbear of second year. Boring. Confusing. Soul-destroying. I'd just grasp one concept and, bam! Another tornado of academic jargon swept it away. Brain. Paralysis.

'Meg, our results have come through!' Bea said, planting a flat palm on my shoulder. 'I've passed, thank God!' she added, throwing her hand over her face in dramatic relief. My stomach flipped. My face flushed. My mind sprinted straight to the vision of me, thirty-five, still working in the garden centre, potting geraniums and sobbing into the compost. I opened the results page and sent up a prayer to whatever deity specialises in academic mercy.

'A fourteen!' I blurted. 'That's a C, right?'

Bea nodded, grinning. Cue celebration. We danced around her uni room like two kids hopped up on Haribo. I even picked up my iPad and planted a kiss on it like a giddy tech worshipper.

'We should go out for tea!' Bea beamed.

'Thought you'd never ask!' I flung my arms in the air and shimmied like a budget drag queen.

We headed to Harvester, celebrating our achievement.

'A pass is a pass, right?' I raised my glass of lemonade. Bea clinked hers of Diet Coke.

'Cheers to that,' she smiled. While we waited for our food, we made a little list of fun things to do when uni wasn't devouring our souls:

- Car karaoke
- Lemon cake and Diet Coke by the sea in summer
- Anything that didn't involve citing sources in Harvard style

Just as we were starting to relax, Bea's phone buzzed with a new message.

'Oh, what's this now?' she frowned. 'Angel said her feedback doesn't match her grade.'

'I haven't even looked at mine yet,' I said, already regretting the decision to open it. We both caved to curiosity and pulled up our essays. Little comment bubbles littered the margins like academic landmines.

'She said my title was too long?' Bea blinked. 'Andi literally told me it was fine when I asked her,' she announced, confused.

'That's jokes,' I laughed. 'Don't worry, Bea, my first comment just says: 'basic introduction' Like... sorry for not writing War and Peace in the opening paragraph.' We scrolled on past the usual 'Good' and 'Could expand on this' until we reached the grand finale: the summary feedback. Bea's was decent, some constructive points, but overall complimentary. Mine? 'Good effort, but you have included lots of research articles that are simply irrelevant; therefore, you lost the reader.' *Simply irrelevant.* I stared at the screen, my appetite evaporating faster than my will to live. I'd spent two months on that essay. Two months of hunting for 'robust literature,' battling with databases, and desperately trying to sound intelligent without actually being intelligent. Bea couldn't stop laughing at the expression on my face.

'Simply irrelevant?' I repeated. 'Charming. That's the name of my autobiography now.'

As if on cue, the waitress arrived with our food. Well, Bea's food.

'I'm so sorry,' she said, flustered. 'The chef missed your order on the ticket. We're getting it sorted now.' Of course they did. Bea and I reassured her it was fine, but honestly? I was done. Nothing had gone straightforwardly lately. And now I had two things in common with the research articles I'd so painstakingly sourced. Simply irrelevant.

CHAPTER

Thirty-Seven

LLANID-LOSING MY MIND

PART ONE

Easter half-term finally came around, and I felt incredibly thankful for some welcomed flexibility in my studying timetables. I had time to sit and read something not to do with giving intravenous benzylpenicillin or teicloplanin. I'd been enjoying reading a novel in the bath the other day, when Mum shouted up, 'Cynthia's on!', a reply to a question from earlier. But my midwifery-wired brain misheard it as 'Syntocinon'. I immediately started planning IV protocols. There was no escape. I ducked under the water in despair. I then spiralled into a deep thought of how I am, in essence, only a bunch of cells walking around the planet. Therefore, is this all worth it, and what is life like now? My heart started to race, and I shot out of the bath only a few minutes after getting in, leaving my existential crisis drain through the plug hole.

Clearly in need of a restorative break, Mum and Dad had decided to book a fancy tent for us to go glamping in Mid-Wales for a few nights during the Easter half-term week. The day soon rolled around quickly, and at eleven o'clock, two hours after her planned departure time, Mum appeared flustered at my door. She was wearing blue jeans and a white hoodie with the slogan 'Spread Happiness', on the front. Her blonde hair was swirled and held in place with a crocodile clip at the back of her head, leaving the ends sticking up where the clip wasn't long enough to grip it. We called it her little fountain.

'Lovely!' She said, relieved as she found me awake. In bed, but awake at least, I gave her a thumbs up and rolled out of bed. My head spun as I'd only opened my eyes three minutes before Mum's appearance. I shoved a jumper on and staggered out of my room and into the hallway. I was greeted by the scene of Mum trying to reason with Joe, who needed reminding that trying to pack his Xbox into an overnight bag for two nights in the Welsh countryside probably wasn't the best use of his space. Joe, a lanky teenager who was already getting close to six feet tall, felt that the best way to avoid this issue was to put the Xbox on his top shelf. Mum was just five foot five.

'You best give that to me,' Mum instructed firmly. 'Right now!'

'But I want to take it, Mum!' Joe retorted.

'For the last time,' she huffed, 'there won't be any electricity for a start; your X-box won't just run on thin air!' Mum explained. Again.

Meanwhile, Al was winding up Marsh, who was easily entertained by the simplest things at only four years young, this time, by my shoelace. Brilliant. Al was wafting the said shoelace in front of the dog's face and whipping it back each time he attempted to claim it with his mouth. I turned around to head back to my room to finish packing from the night before, but Al's laughter drew my attention back to the fact my shoelace now had a Dalmatian hanging off the end of it and the more I tried to get it back it seemed more of it disappeared.

'Marsh, stop it!' I tried to tug it from him. 'Spit it out! Come on, Marsh,' I said with a smile, trying to reason with him, and he finally spat it out. Unimpressed, I flung the regurgitated, slobbery shoelace onto the stairs, past the gate and out of his reach. I stood up, my hair on end and most of the dog's white hair littering my black jumper. Al continued to laugh and mocked my 'minging' shoelace, which flopped sadly on the stairs whilst she was putting on her brand new, white trainers that cost her two hundred and fifty quid. I wonder how she'd cope if I fed her shoelaces to the dog. It would probably cost thirty quid a chew.

Thirty minutes later, Dad's arms sunk with the weight of my life smashed into my overnight bag as he stuffed it into the car for me. We left fifteen minutes later after unlocking and re-locking the house four times for forgotten essentials: a non-itchy picnic blanket, a third charger, another West Ham top, and a jumper free of dalmatian confetti. At long last, the house was locked; all five of us in the car and leaving the driveway. 12.34, three hours and thirty-four minutes later than planned. We only made it to the second street before Dad turned us back around as he, too, had forgotten something important: his sunglasses. It was raining and forecast for storms. We all huffed and puffed as he insisted. The poor dog was confused by the end of it, watching us back and forth like a little game of ping pong.

'Ty Llywellyn' marked our destination deep in rural Welsh terrain. It was a long but pleasant drive, journeying through the emerald countryside.

'It says we call her when we get to the entrance, and she'll meet us here,' Mum said after Dad had gone around in a loop.

'I'm sure I can find my way alright without any help,' Dad spat out, classically defending his independence even though no one questioned it in the first place. Al and Mum simultaneously sighed while Joe and I remained on the fence. Mum broke the tension apart by ringing the phone number provided, and I knew we all knew we were in for another delay. Mum had a knack for talking on the phone, and it remains a talent to this day. Given how long it took for us to move a few hours up the country, we were going to arrive at the time of checkout at that rate.

'Right, she's making her way over with her sons, Ben and Levi, now,' Mum said happily many minutes later. I love how she knew her kids' names after the first phone call; I'd be calling her Auntie Sarah by the time we got to the tent. Joe and his motoring radar sprung into action as he heard an engine popping in the distance. He swivelled around to the direction of its origin, with his face pressed against the window to examine it holistically. Al and I exchanged a smile.

'She's riding a quad, Mum!' Joe announced. 'Although a bit of a shit one, I can't lie,' he added under his breath as it drew closer. A woman wearing jeans, long brown boots and a checkered shirt supported herself off the quad. She walked with a heavy swagger, like her back pockets were full of bricks, her legs wide apart, boots thudding across the ground. I marvelled over her powerful stance as she came to a halt and shoved her hands in her back pockets. 'Croeso i chi', she beamed at us all. 'Welcome to you all'.

Sarah led us further into the valley's crease, where green fields stretched over the landscape with only three tents dotted on the landscape. I squinted to make out a flock of sheep as tiny white specs scattered randomly across the mountainside. It was so Welsh, I loved it. Perched tightly on a large mound of mud, stones sat comfortably around it; Sarah led us to a circus-like tent with an outdoor kitchen to the left and a shower cubicle and a bath tucked behind it on the right. I couldn't help but notice that, as quickly as Al did, it looked small. I wondered if it would be like Harry Potter, where it expands to something three times the size once you go in. Sarah, Mum and Dad brought up their conversation about amenities, facilities, and all the other essential 'ities' that there were to know, whereby by the end, she said she must get on to tend to her hen that's struggling with constipation. Of course, she did. Mum mentioned I was training to be a midwife, and Sarah asked me if she could give laxatives to a chicken. I evaded any sort of responsibility by saying I wasn't allowed to recommend anything, wasn't close to qualifying, plus the most sensible answer would be to absolutely not give your chicken a human laxative. I couldn't help thinking of this poor chicken shitting out an egg every few minutes. Maybe that was the aim? Like a poorly evidenced business ploy.

'Well, thank you. I will see you later on,' Sarah wobbled over to the quad and plonked herself on the edge while her five-year-old smashed his foot on the accelerator and drove them unsteadily away. I glanced to see Joe in a trance of amazement.

'Right here we go', Dad said excitedly as he took the lead to enter the yurt. Our suspicions of a small tent were confirmed; a blue two-seated settee was near the entrance, which also concealed a double bed behind it. My attention was instantly stolen by a central fireplace. Hold up. I brought my eyes back to a fire in a tent. Trying not to think about whether Sarah was going to find us all dead by carbon monoxide poisoning come morning, my mind was soon brought back to the present moment as Dad sat on the sofa with a questionable sound from its stability. He sat proudly in his pink polo shirt and flashed us all a smile of 'I'm on annual leave, and I don't care what it's like', which was fair enough. After we had photographed the moment, we all eventually piled in, squabbling around and trying not to knock each other out. We were all a lot bigger than the last time we went camping. Joe especially, almost as tall as me at the age of fourteen, had a slender build which made his hands look like small dinner plates. Al, on the other hand, is five feet tall, small, and athletic. That only left me different again; curvy, they would say and not of the 'athletic' or 'slender' description like my fellow siblings.

'Mum. Not being funny, but where are we going to sleep?' Al gestured to exhibit A and B of the double bed only. To be fair to her, I wondered where C, D and E would sleep too. A family discussion broke out, and we all talked over each other and tried to devise solutions to the issue. Joe was in the background, his hand covering his entire face; Dad fixated on measuring the interior's sturdiness; Mum took the positive approach, and Al batted off the positivity with her racquet of realism.

'Where am I physically going to sleep, though?' Al pushed. 'I ain't sleeping on the floor with my knee; nah, you're joking!' She shook her head in rejection as Mum tried to diffuse her. I realised my suggestion fell on deaf ears, so instead, I rummaged around and soon figured out that Dad was sitting on a sofa bed, which made it able to sleep four. We were still a family of five, though, Auntie Sarah. Where would our fifth member sleep? Joe passed through the corner of my eye as he left the noise of the rest of us behind, exiting the tent. I caught a glimpse of him as I peered through the entrance. He stood at the edge of the mud mound, looking out onto the rolling hills in the distance. Despite being only fourteen, I realised how much he had grown lately; he looked at least nineteen. Innocent and gentle, Joe was seen as precious to us all. It was nice to watch him chilling, comfortable in his own company and able to soak up the atmosphere. I saw his shadow look the tent up and down and loudly but somewhat calmly groan to the skies.

'Well, this is shit,' piercing the precious bubble I'd built around him.

After a lot of family commotion, failed phone calls and more commotion, we discovered that Sarah had put airbeds in one of the cupboards for us. We finally escaped the situation and decided to walk into the town. It was supposedly a ten-minute stroll to the pub, but someone somewhere definitely couldn't measure time, or they flew there because it took a lot longer than ten minutes. The only signs pointing toward the pub seemed to submerge us into the woods and eventually another spindly lane. I swivelled around to try and see where the actual hell we were. Dad joined me, looking into the distance, screwed his nose up and dropped his mouth open; the infamous concentration face. Al silently pointed to a sign: 'Mulberry Farm, private land, NO entry, guns on the property, trespassers cross at own risk'. Was that a joke? Guns on their property. My mind immediately flicked to the concept of farmers being legally allowed to shoot anyone and anything on their land at any given time.

'Trespassing my land, Meg!' She shouted playfully with a tinge of aggression.

'Guns? What?' Joe questioned bluntly. We were having an audible panic in the middle of a lane we were not supposed to be in, and as a result, we were drawing attention to ourselves. Mum clocked on and shot a look Al's way, which she received well.

'Sorry,' She said sarcastically. 'Sorry, he can't handle a sign.' Maybe she didn't receive it quite so well after all. Dad decided to interject and led the family pack in the other direction. Mum tried to calm Joe, and I joked with Al about how Sarah may be just as full of shit as her chicken when she gave us those directions.

'Excuse me, excuse me!' Said an unfamiliar voice. We all turned in sync to see a tall woman standing a few feet away. Her blonde hair swept the shoulder straps of her denim dungarees. My vision was almost right. As she drew closer, it was apparent she was holding something. We were all on edge after what we had read, not moments before this. As she came into focus, we realised she had a baby resting on her hip, not a shotgun. Every cloud and its silver lining, as they say. I tried to show Joe, but he did not have any of it. He just refused to look at anything other than the floor. Although I relaxed when I saw she was with a child and not a weapon, she still very impolitely told us to clear off, despite Mum's best efforts to apologise. We exited the lane and ended up back to where we started. Brilliant. Joe slumped behind my parents as they tried to decipher which route to take next. Dad tried to regain a bar by stretching his hand up towards the clouds as if asking for a bit of help from God. God didn't decide to help him out that day, and we lost the signal totally and ended up wading our way through the stingy nettles that dominated the road. After a lot of perseverance, we finally reached the pub; no lights on, and was boarded up shut.

'Fuck,' I mouthed silently.

'Nah, this is an actual joke,' Al said and crossed her arms. What was supposed to be a ten-minute walk turned into a survival trek through the Welsh wilderness. Two of us cried, three of us were threatened by a woman with dungarees, and five out of five got stung by nettles. We all arrived back with one shared conclusion: happy half-term, my arse.

PART TWO

After we finally returned home from our outing, everyone got to what they could do best; Dad unpacked the car and handed everything to Mum to position in her way. Al carped at the side, her arms crossed over her stomach, shielding her small frame from the cold. Joe set up the fire pit and tossed anything he could find into the budding flames. I moved back over to the view but noticed he had gotten hold of a 'prodder', as we called it at home. But this time, it seemed to have caught fire. He twirled it like the Olympic torch, which instantly caught Dad's attention.

'Umm, Joey, please be careful with that. You need to put it out,' Mum's voice shook slightly whilst Dad just glared at the unfolding situation.

'It's fine, Mum; it's only small,' he squinted as he pulled the item rather close to his face to get a better look.

'Joe, not too close to your face, yeah? You'll be without a nose in a minute,' she paused. 'Have you got your contacts in?' She asked with a touch of concern.

'No, took them out so I can see the fire better,' he replied, deadly serious. Did I hear that right? I realised he was serious and turned my attention to Mum, anticipating her response.

'I'm shocked you can't see it at all, Joe. You need them on to see what you're doing when you play with fire!' As serious as she was, laughter managed to escape her. As she always did, something I've always admired is that there is a reason to laugh. Even if Joe was about to practice stop, drop and roll.

After the drama of assessing the likelihood of my brother burning his facial features off and the entire place down (then we really wouldn't have anywhere to sleep), I found myself rather intrigued by the prospect of having a warm bath in the outdoors, and here was my opportunity. I announced that I was about to change into my swimming costume, restricting access to the tent for five minutes. I quickly changed as I didn't trust they would have adequately listened or cared enough to retain the information.

The thought of them seeing me naked motivated me to a speedy change. Comfortably insulated in the warm water, I cast my eyes to the view ahead of me. I looked out onto the hills and witnessed the sun strolling slowly across the sky's lower end. It left a pretty orange glow behind it. Eventually, it faded out of my sight and made way for a sprinkle of silver stars to come into focus in its place. I inhaled a deep breath, to which I smelt the smell of Joe's blind fire, and my ears absorbed the voices of my people, at which point I closed my eyes and switched off from life for a while and bloody hell did it feel good. It was one of the first times I appreciated mindfulness and considered its importance for sustaining positive mental health.

Everyone started settling for the night by about eleven o'clock, given that we had had a long day. I climbed onto my handmade bed from the sofa, which resembled a brick wall; only this one was coated in blue velvet, but a brick wall, nonetheless. As I led there, I looked up and saw a black spider from which I immediately fled my brick wall and shouted that a spider was residing up there and that I would certainly not be alongside it.

'Ugh, nah, I'm not sleeping next to that,' Al spat out in pure disgust. Dad sighed, as he didn't believe squashing them was kind. However, he clearly decided it would be in his favour to do as we all wished here and squished it to restore our sanities. Joe finally clocked on, about three years after the first spider had met its end.

'I'm not spending my time here tonight with his family,' he insisted, shaking his head.

'It's fine it's gone now, I wouldn't be sleeping in here if there were any more, Joe,' I said confidently. It was as if the spider in question's arachnid clan was indeed listening, and Joe spotted another one dangling from the drawers in the corner. How could he spot that but not see the fire earlier? It made me believe he had selective sight problems when it suited him.

'Aghh Meg, there's another one crawling over there,' Al raised her voice from the other side of the tent. Nothing seemed to be straightforward.

'Right bloody hell, where's my slipper gone? And you get that one, and I'll get this one.' Mum decided to take charge of the situation. She released her teacher's side. Nevertheless, Dad was still sitting on the bed with his arms resting beneath his head, trying to deflect the situation onto insect rights.

'Imagine if someone killed Meg,' he said randomly.

'Thanks a bunch, Dad. It's nice to know I'm the first one you think of when you think of who would be most likely to get killed,' I laughed.

'Then they killed you and Joe, too,' he changed the audience of his comment to Al as she looked at him with utter disapproval. 'How do you think Mum and I would feel?' He gave us a rhetorical.

‘Piss off And, I’ll get it my frigging self,’ Mum fumed as she charged around the bed and Dad got out on his side to evict the other. ’Right, all gone now; everyone can settle down now,’ Mum extinguished the situation. Before we had a moment to retaliate, a great, hairy one sprinted from under the bed and past me, to which Al and I freaked out. We shot out of the tent shouting loudly and was quickly accompanied by a shaky Joe who later offered to torch the place as a solution. We all stood outside the tent, shivering as the cold air wrapped around our bodies and lungs. We stood there in silence, exhaling white swirls of warm air into the already cool night sky. I slung an arm around Joe’s growing shoulders and pulled him close. We stood there in the dark, exhaling white breath into the night sky. For a second, it felt like the whole world had paused for us. Just a brother and two sisters, silently bonded by mutual spider trauma.

The serenity was cut short when we heard the sound of Mum slapping her slipper multiple times. Al and I twisted our eyebrows into complete concern.

‘Ummm, Mum, what’s going on in there?’ I proceed to ask with a nervous smile. Before she even got the chance to answer, I heard a few more slaps. Convinced my parents were winding me up, I untangled myself from Joe and peered through the tent flap. I popped my head in slightly, only to see Mum kneeling on the floor. I sniggered, but they didn’t even twitch; then I noticed Mum was enclosed in multiple splats of brown. She was poised with her fluffy crimson slider above her shoulder, anticipating her next action of defence. My peripheral vision watched Dad as he reached far up the flimsy walls of the adjacent side of the yurt. I realised he was aiming for another huge spider. A genuine infestation. Brilliant.

I rejoined my siblings outside, and for the next twenty minutes, all we could see was the shadows of our parents slapping multiple objects. No other tents were slapping their furniture. Mum finally emerged from the tent. Her hair looked like she'd been given some bad news; red cheeks and cradling a bunch of tissues. She looked at us all with a tired expression as she emptied the contents of her arms into the black bin.

'Not going to lie to you kids, there's been at least twenty spiders in there,' she admitted. Our faces dropped. The only sound was the soft buzz of the wildlife across the valley.

'Bloody glamping,' she said in frustration.

'Come on, Al and Joe, I'll set you guys up in the car,' she shuffled them along. 'Meg, can you cope in the tent?' She asked hopefully. I nodded, desperate for the ordeal to be over. But I hated spiders. Really hated them. I pulled the duvet over my head and created a literal cocoon around me. I found myself tossing and turning, attempting to get off to sleep, but without success.

I drifted off for a little while but woke to find my watch illuminated with 02.34 displayed across its screen. Fucks sake. Then, the feeling of needing a wee washed over me. I reached for my phone and pressed the torch icon, which blinded me with a flash of white light. I cast it over the tent with a suspicious mind. However, I couldn't see anything, suggesting I was in the clear. I crept out barefoot, tiptoeing over the stones, until I hit a loose patch and skidded straight downhill, flailing like a broken windmill. My arms and legs were splayed out in all sorts of weird angles. I couldn't control the speed of my fall and smashed myself against the car, rocking it a tad. Great for the self-esteem. My face was squished against the window, and I noticed Al and Joe fast asleep, top to tail. I sighed, which fogged up the window and obstructed my view of them. I was glad they managed to get to sleep. I pressed both of my hands against the window and pushed, peeling my face off of the window.

PART THREE

As soon as the sun gave rise to a new day, we all gathered outside to eat breakfast. With the rising sun, Al and Joe sang praises for the car as a place to rest their heads. Lucky them. Gladly, we had a more successful day; we found our way to the local reservoir and watched red kites soar above it. We found an open pub and had a lovely meal before returning to the tent for the evening. As the second day transitioned to dusk, I decided it was time I had another bath. I decided this time I would go commando, though, as my swimming costume was three sizes too small for me I felt like an enlarged pig in a blanket with how tight it was and where I was popping out. Plus, no one could view us from the outside as there was a steep hill behind us, and we were the furthest tent, so no one would need to walk past. I headed over to the bath and evaluated the area around me. Not another human to be seen. Perfect.

I led down and submerged myself underneath the bubbles. I squirmed around to try and find the most comfortable position. With boobs the size of Jupiter and Saturn, naturally, they floated to the surface like a pair of rescue buoys. I looked like I'd survived a shipwreck, chest first. Rolling with my own force of nature, I closed my eyes and enjoyed being free in the water, even if my boobs were fulfilling their role as bobbing apples at Halloween. After nearly ten minutes, my phone buzzed. It was Al, so I hung over the side of the bath. Jupiter was hanging outside of the tub with me, and I awkwardly fumbled for my phone. I answered it and heard Al advising me to abort my plan and commence plan b as a family of adults and kids made their way up towards our tent. Bollocks. I also found the bubbles had disintegrated, and you could literally see every part of me through the transparent water.

I had no words. I peered around the corner, and low and behold, a group of people were hiking up and getting dangerously close to our yurt. Why though? Immediately after that thought, a memory found its way to the forefront of my mind. I recall Sarah explaining that you can see spectacular views from the top of the hill. Particularly on a clear night at about dusk. Double bollocks. I started to panic but tried to find some rationalism in it. I couldn't get up as that was literally asking for them to stare. But then I couldn't stay there either as my boobs were practically giving the morse code a run for its money. I scanned for options. There were none. Then came the torches, bright white beams scanning across the hill like searchlights. What happened to the hill being our natural privacy screen? Suddenly, it was centre stage. Their voices grew louder. Closer. I panicked, flattened my boobs against my chest, and slid backwards, completely submerging myself. I couldn't see, breathe, or hear. Brilliant. Slowly, I rose back up out of the water, just my nose and eyes exposed like a pervy submarine. I felt like James Bond, if James Bond had tits and a crippling fear of being seen by strangers.

'Meg, it's me,' Mum's voice called out. 'You alright? There are some people standing right above you looking ou- wait... are those your boobs?' Her eyebrows shot up so high I thought they might launch off her face entirely. I lifted my mouth above the surface. 'Yes, Mum. I can confirm, they are, indeed, my boobs.' I glanced down. Two nipples, standing to attention. One pointing east. The other west. Me in the middle, floating in existential shame.

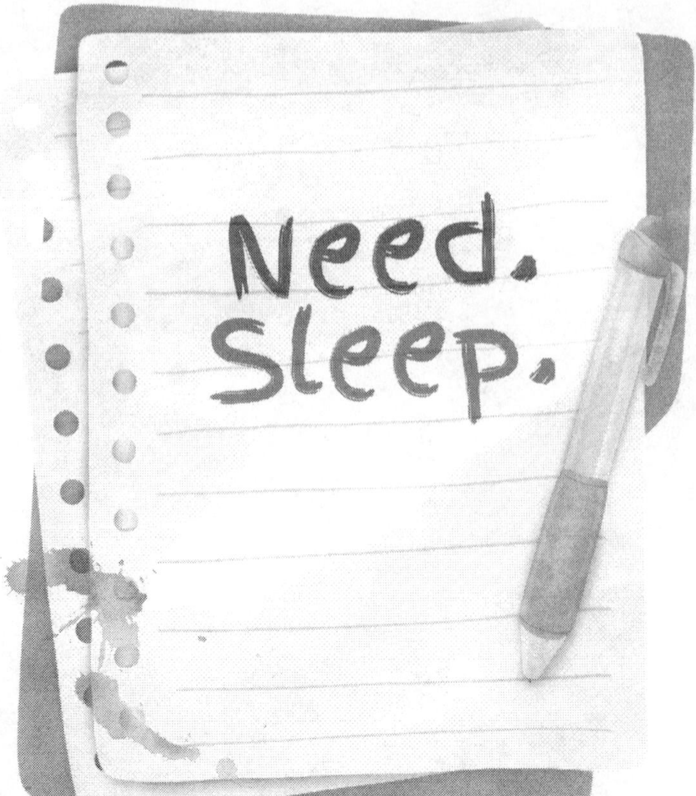
Need.
Sleep.

CHAPTER
Thirty-Eight

A THREE-COURSE DISASTER

After surviving the wild world of glamping, university resumed with another theory block, because nothing says 'welcome back' like academic whiplash. Our lecturers had a real talent for squeezing three months of chaos into three weeks. A gift, really. One wrapped in existential dread. This time, we did two presentations, launched a new essay (a few days after the last was submitted) and dived headfirst into the complexities of obstetric emergencies. One day, in particular, comes to mind when eclamptic seizures, shoulder dystocia and cord prolapse were on the menu. Brutal. Although I couldn't help but wish they had taught us this *before* I had a run-in with them on the last placement. Regardless, it was another three-course itinerary of all things terrifying and a big wake-up call to the sheer responsibility of being a midwife.

First course: eclamptic seizures. Caused by severe pre-eclampsia, formally known as Pre-Eclampsia Toxaemia (hence the abbreviation PET, and as we all know by now, not the gerbil kind). It all made sense now. PET occurs when high blood pressure wreaks havoc on a pregnant body, pushing it to breaking point. It's still one of obstetrics' most misunderstood conditions, symptoms that sound like either pregnancy or something horrendous: swelling, headaches, blurred vision, upper abdominal pain. Are we putting banners out to say welcome to your new pregnant body or to the PET party? Your job? Work out which. Hence why, we jump straight on you when you present us with some cheeky symptoms of PET and given that PET is like a chameleon hiding in plain sight, it arguably makes it one of the most dangerous conditions of all. Interestingly, you're more likely to have PET in your first pregnancy, coupled with a family history of the condition, smoking, but let's be honest, smoking is just a fast-track pass for all things dangerous in life and particularly obstetrics whilst simultaneously emptying your bank account. What's the point?

Following the bitter taste of PET, we moved on to the main course, Shoulder Dystocia (SD). Unlike PET, SD is much more objective and easier to comprehend. A baby's shoulders essentially get stuck during a vaginal birth. They get stuck behind, most commonly, the symphysis pubis (that little bone just under the bikini line) or, less commonly, the sacrum of the pelvis. Either way, once the head has birthed, ideally, we should have the rest of the baby on the next contraction or two. If that doesn't happen, we have an SD and five minutes to get that baby out before we enter territory for severe compromise for the baby. The weight of responsibility started weighing heavy on my own shoulders at this point. Did I even want this responsibility? First up: the McRoberts position; knees to ears. It widens the pelvis and gives the baby more wiggle room. Amazingly, this alone fixes the issue in up to ninety percent of cases. If not, we go external: suprapubic pressure, pressing just above the pubic bone to squeeze the shoulders inward. Still stuck? Then it's time to fish for an arm, posterior, always. Because if the baby can't get through, good luck to your hand at the anterior entry.

I found the SD lecture too heavy for my liking and would have left the hypothetical restaurant if I had a choice. Sadly, I was obliged to have dessert. Dessert, unfortunately not an apple pie, but cord prolapse. If the umbilical cord comes out first, it gets squashed by the baby on its way down. Bad news. That cord is their life source. No oxygen is big trouble. The solution? A crash caesarean. But until then, someone, usually the midwife, has to keep their hand inside, lifting the baby off their own cord. It's ridiculous, heroic, and a logistical nightmare. Occasionally, the midwife goes to theatre too, crouched between legs, praying not to sneeze.

The weight of all this responsibility followed me everywhere. I found myself thinking about eclamptic seizures in the shower, running shoulder dystocia manoeuvres in the Sainsbury's queue, mentally elevating imaginary babies in traffic. All this, for fifteen pounds an hour. It didn't exactly scream 'bargain.' A few weeks later, after a hellish shift, I cried, shock. One woman had a UPCR (test for PET) of

1020 (diagnosis threshold: thirty). Another was talked into induction over a supposedly 'big baby' and the risk of SD (despite evidence being wooly). A third claimed something was hanging out of her vagina, turns out, just mucous. Never thought cervical slime could trigger a cardiac event. I was twenty. My friends were building businesses, launching apps, conquering adult life. Me? I was elbow-deep in bodily fluids, doubting everything. Hello, imposter syndrome. Everything I did, somehow midwifery would weave its way in. I guess it was the subconscious pressure of one day having literally both mum and baby's life in your hands at all times. I wondered horribly if I was really up to the task in hand or not...

CHAPTER
Thirty-Nine

THE TRIALS OF TRIAGE

Following that heavy theory block, we were released back into clinical practice. Once again, in X, I made my way to triage, which was nothing other than a baptism of fire. With the number of baptisms of fires I had experienced over the last six years, I was surprised I wasn't burnt to a crisp.

'Morning Meg, you ready for it again?' Jo asked brightly. Jo was one of the most amazing mentors I had the pleasure of working with. She was wildly knowledgeable and had a stentorian way of advocating for those in her care. She made patients, me, and her cat feel like we could do anything. She was exactly as ace as she sounded and exactly what my panicked brain needed after dealing with the polar opposite.

'Yes, Jo, right here with you!' I beamed back, pretending I wasn't shitting it. It was the truly unexpected elements of triage that I wasn't a massive fan of, regardless of the mentor.

'Meg, you look worried. Is anything on your mind?' She asked, having a fully accurate read on me.

'Ahh yeah, I just find myself jumped up by this place at the moment, overthinking every symptom,' I exhaled with some relief from speaking my uneasy mind. 'Literally, the night before last, a woman came in with a headache, I had a headache, too, and I was convinced we were both about to die from PET,' I laughed. I wasn't even pregnant, and she told us she hadn't slept for a day and a half, and funnily enough, a little paracetamol and little sleep did the trick...

'Honestly, Meg, you're doing a good job; the more shifts you have, the better it will be,' she said nicely. Jo said I worried too much, but I recognised I was overcompensating after Sandra, Rhian and co humiliated me.

Jo ducked behind the desk to find a long-lost pen or something, and I took a moment to look out of the window into the world. The little area stood still with the warmth of the spring air sitting nicely. I took a long breath and reminded myself that I wasn't with Sandra; it was a different midwife, a different day, and a different set of patients.

'So, in bed one, a woman is waiting for a doctor review following a PV* bleed,' she pointed at the following, 'bed two, reduced movements, we need to do everything obs, CTG, and go from there.' She tapped on the door buzzer to let another couple in. 'Bed three is in for a CTG after a midwife heard a deceleration in community, bed four is just being cleaned, and bed five is supposed to be for a labourer that called at four o'clock,' she flicked to her fob watch, 'which was four hours ago now so we will call them in a bit and see what's going on,' she said casually.

'Right,' I exhaled. 'Shall I start with bed two?' I asked for confirmation. Jo nodded, and we dispersed into the lives of complete strangers.

I found bed two housed a lady called Nicole; first baby, thirty weeks and even after a few moments of knowing her, I realised she was terrified of something bad happening to her baby as she'd waited five long years for this pregnancy. One thing about midwifery I enjoyed so far was seeing the relief on faces when I could reassure them or even provide support if it wasn't going well. The art of making a minute difference fed my desire to practice.

'Can I ask a silly question, Meg, please?' She asked with longing in her eyes as I strapped the CTG monitor in place to hear the familiar beat of her baby's heartbeat.

'Of course you can. Nothing is silly, and if I can't answer it, I will find someone who can,' I implored.

'Will red socks give off bad energy to the baby?' She looked genuinely worried. 'I read about the colour red being superstitious for the unborn population once, and now I'm worried bad vibes might get to him,' she looked almost nauseous at the thought. Thankfully, I was able to provide reassurance by confirming that her baby couldn't give a toss about the colour of her socks and that there was no evidence of bad vibes when travelling from red socks to the unborn. Although I delivered it much more sensitively and professionally. What made me laugh to myself was that she seemed to be more reassured by the busting of the red sock myth over a completely normal CTG and obs and that her baby was moving by the time she left triage. Jo was happy too with how I 'gracefully handled the red sock situation and treated it like any other question,' which I took in my stride. It left me feeling a little buzz for what was next, keen to impress my mentor and help X's pregnant population in any way I could. Super Meg energy. Here. We. Go.

Bed three, Cheryl, thirty-seven weeks, continued to have decelerations. She was contracting but even still, after a while the decelerations were classed as late, which, for her, started after the peak of her contractions and were slow to recover, making them one of our more pathological kinds. Therefore, she was transferred to Delivery Suite for further management and probable delivery if it continued and her cervix remained at one centimetre as it was at the time. Cheryl, however, didn't seem to worry herself and asked me if she could go home to get her slippers first. Sometimes, we couldn't even solve a pathological CTG trace without a caesarean section, let alone a pair of fluffy slippers, so funnily enough, the answer was no. She accepted and got straight on the phone to ask her partner Nas if he could bring her slippers as she would be 'staying in for a bit'. I admired her calmness regardless of the reason.

Bed one, Mickaela, told me that her bleeding occurred after having sex and asked if they should be worried about conceiving another baby or not? Again, I was able to provide reassurance of a definite no to simultaneous conception when you are already six months deep. When I got them settled on the maternity ward for the night, they seemed relieved and thanked me profusely for my help. I practically skipped back to triage as the patient seemed grateful for the knowledge I was sharing with them, and clearly, for me, things were finally falling into place; where theoretical midwifery and practical midwifery were understanding each other, not just talking to each other in different languages...

'Okay, can I speak to your wife, or can you put me on speaker?' Jo asked in an instructive tone I didn't hear unless something was going on. I looked over to her as I cleared up after another lady had come and gone for query SROM (spontaneous rupture of membranes, i.e. amniotic fluid most of us refer to as waters). They had definitely gone as I was still mopping up puddles after she'd left almost half an hour ago.

'Okay, if you think the baby is going to be born soon and you can't get in the car to come to us, we will have to call an ambulance,' Jo said sternly. 'Okay, wait, so contractions have stopped now?' She asked, as confused as I felt. I stretched over the bed to sweep the top of it clean, and at that moment, I turned to catch a glimpse of a man banging the doors, pleading for help. I abandoned my Clinell wipes, hopped over the mop and clambered to the door.

'What's wrong? How can I help?' I asked as I swung the door open.

'My wife, bleeding,' he said in a thick Eastern European accent laced with panic.

'Okay, where is she?' I asked, as I couldn't place any eyes on her.

'In corridor,' he answered plainly although, I couldn't see anyone in the long, dark corridor other than him. Was it a game of prank the midwife instead of call the midwife?

'Jo, sorry, a woman bleeding somewhere. Can I go and investigate, or do you want me to stay?' I asked as Jo had thankfully just put down the phone receiver.

'Ahh, Jesus, okay, Meg,' she put her hand on her forehead and sighed elongatedly. I'll go, you stay; tell Delivery Suite you're on your own for a minute, just in case,' she picked up a pair of gloves and shoved them into her pocket. 'If the phone goes, open a triage assessment on the computer, do your best, put her on hold, and I will run it over with you when I'm back,' she said quickly.

'Okay, sure,' I nodded, wondering how one person could handle this solo. Jo quickly disappeared into the shadows, and I was left with an eerie darkness as two o'clock flashed on the computer screen. I'd given Delivery Suite a call but had no answer. Charming. Five minutes into my lone spell on triage, the phone started ringing in its dulcet tone. An external number, a real person, shit. Open her record. Do your best. Jo will be back. I psyched myself up, letting the phone ring at me for another two tones before eventually picking it up.

'Hello, maternity triage X, Megan speaking,' I addressed the unknown caller.

'I called earlier, but I think it's happening now. She's on the floor and pushing, maybe?' a man with a shaky voice said. Shit! I asked for her record and pulled it up to find this was her third baby. Triple shit.

'Daviiiiiid,' a voice in the background shouted.

'Have you called an ambulance, David?' I asked with urgency.

'Yeah, but they said to try and get to the hospital if we have time as there are no crews available,' he said plainly. Before I had a chance to reply, I heard another almighty scream in the background. 'Wait, I think I can see some of the baby!' he explained. Some of the baby? Tell me there's hair. God, let it be hair, not a foot or anything else, which would make both David's and my job a whole lot harder.

'David put me on speaker, please,' I said instructively, as Jo always did when she meant business. I pressed a call bell to try to alert one of the midwives from elsewhere, but again, no one came. I'd like to take this moment to thank X's Delivery Suite for their continued support (or lack of) throughout my training.

'Hello, Michelle! I hear you're doing a fantastic job. My name is Meg, and I'm going to help you through this!' I tried to say as calmly as I could.

'It's coming out of me!' She screamed.

'I can see a bit of hair, I think, God, what do I do?' David alluded to panic. I instructed him to get some towels at the ready while I dialled for an ambulance on the other phone. After a very brief conversation with the operation handler, they were going to dispatch an ambulance as soon as possible, but in my heart of hearts, I knew there wouldn't be time for that.

'Michelle, breathe. Your baby is ready to meet you. All seems normal from what you've told me, and David can see, too,' I reassured her. Michelle let out a compulsive wail as I envisioned her baby's head edging its way out.

'Christ alive, it's getting bigger and bigger!' David exclaimed.

'Shut up, you knobhead!' Michelle spat. 'AGHHHH!' She screamed again. If I hadn't been so stressed, I would have cracked a smile, but even I didn't have time for humour.

'Breathe, Michelle. It's important to do small pushes at this stage. I know it seems impossible, but try and do what you can,' I replied when Jo came back to triage with the bleeding lady who had just lazily strolled into bed space one. Thankfully, she was not so bleedy after all. Jo whipped the curtain around and came to me immediately, her features stretched in curiosity as she skimmed through the woman's record and my notes so far.

'IT'S FUCKING COMING OUT OF ME!' Michelle screamed.

'David, put your hands gently on baby's head, ready to greet them. Michelle, breathe for me. Little push now!' Jo's face turned a different shade, and I was afraid she was going to grab the phone and tell me I was a disaster, but instead, she smiled, deciding not to intervene.

'Christ alive, that's quite big actually,' David commented, still in awe of the process.

'FUCK OFF, DAVIDDDD!' Michelle elongated.

'Wait, I can see eyebrows!' David squealed.

'Little push, Michelle. David, support the baby's head now!' Jo continued to smile and listen to the phone that was pinned to my ear.

'Baby's head is out and turning around? Why is it turning around? Is it going back in?'

'It's normal for baby to turn, guys. They are moving their shoulders. Well done, Michelle. Next contraction and baby should be here,' I wiped away a bead of sweat on my brow.

'I literally have our baby in my hands; what the fuck is going on?' He said, stunned. That was me at every birth as a student, the difference being David was allowed to let it out.

'Well done, David, keep supporting baby and keep your towels at the ready.'

'This was not the plan; I liked my cream carpet,' Michelle crescendoed. 'It's coming again!'

'Big push, last push, Michelle!' I encouraged.

'He's so long!' David exclaimed.

'You're telling me!' Michelle boomed.

There was a brief moment of silence followed swiftly by the sound of a little squeak from their baby boy, delivered by his dad, onto their cream carpet at quarter past two in the morning.

'He's okay!' David beamed.

'Oh my God!' Michelle started crying.

'Well done! To Michelle, David. Get those towels over him; congratulations!' I said, listening intently to the baby screaming, a vital sign that he was okay. 'Is he pinking up David? Tell me what he's doing,' I asked.

'He's waving his hands around and looking around at the mess of the carpet, Shelle!' He said with the utmost relief.

'Right, now tell me what Michelle's blood loss is doing David, please.'

'Not much,' he said unsure.

'Describe it to me?' I asked instinctively.

'About a dinner plate size?' David estimated with great thought.

'Perfect, okay,' I grinned as I looked to Jo, who had written down the details of the phone call on the woman's record. She gave me a thumbs-up when I asked what she would have. Gladly, the ambulance crew arrived before the placenta, and I got off the phone at about three with a grateful Michelle and David, who asked to meet me when they arrived like I was a celeb.

'You just delivered a baby over the phone, and beautifully might I add!' Jo beamed as she sat back onto the chair and folded her arms. 'What a night!'

'Can you sign it as part of the forty babies I have to deliver, then, Jo?' She tapped my arm affectionately and winked.

Thankfully, Jo dealt with bed space one while she made me tea and biscuits. Not long ago, I was terrified to speak up in a room of midwives. Now I'd just guided a baby into the world from two postcodes away. Maybe I wasn't just surviving anymore - I was actually doing this. Michelle and David finally arrived at the hospital at about half past three, and I popped over to Delivery Suite to greet them. Thankfully, baby was fine, he frowned at me when I met the little man. Michelle was a small lady with the warmest eyes, and David, tall and lanky, shook my hand vigorously when he put a face to the voice. My veins were pumped with the adrenaline of being a bit of a midwife for the night, even if it was over the phone. I eventually returned to triage to find three more beds occupied and Jo buzzing around, dealing with it all over again. I guess that was the nature of triage; absolutely anyone could call about anything, whether it be red socks, fluffy slippers or birthing on your bedroom floor; it was a consistent escalator of case after case, one extreme to the next.

*meaning Per Vaginal (PV).

CHAPTER

Forty

THE SEVEN-YEAR CURSE

I often spent my sacred days off with my nearest and dearest, usually Bea or my family. So, between another crazy shift on triage where we called two emergency caesarean sections and someone later called about whether it was safe to use Vaseline in pregnancy (talk about two extremes), Grandma and I went off to the garden centre for the day with the plan to unwind with the plants.

Watching the bees buzz around the flowers, with a slither of sun peeking out from the clouds here and there, I felt a million miles away from midwifery. I have recognised that downtime is just as important as work time. Another fundamental lesson of life.

'What's wrong, Meg?' Grandma asked as I stopped in my tracks, mid-gardening glove aisle.

'Is that who I think it is?' I whispered, frozen mid-step in the gardening glove aisle. Grandma squinted. 'Who? The woman by the geraniums?'

'That's Nina's nan,' I said impulsively.

'And?' Grandma looked worried for my welfare.

'She's supposed to be dead, Grandma!'

'She looks pretty good to me?' Grandma enquired worriedly and put her ladybird gloves back on the shelf.

'That's just it, Grandma,' I let out an edgy laugh, 'she looks pretty good for seven years dead!' I whispered severely. Nina, who I met in secondary school and eventually fell out with after a false rumour and a thousand tiny betrayals, was the same Nina who sobbed into my jumper when her nan supposedly died. I even baked her a cake as a sorry for her loss, and we cried on the sofa together watching Gilmore Girls...What in the world was that all about?

'Unless she meant her other nan?' Grandma sensibly offered.

'Well, apparently, her other nan died when she was six, so unless she's about to walk around the corner in a minute for good measure...' I laughed. Whichever way, Nana Heather certainly didn't have her burial; she looked better than I did! As if on cue, Nina's Mum appeared out of nowhere, but at least I expected her to breathe if I saw her again. She looked shifty once she saw me gawping at them and steered her mother in the other direction.

'Maybe she knew more than she let on all those years ago, Meg,' Grandma said sceptically, peering over the top of her glasses like a little inspector.

'You're telling me!' I said as I stared at the empty space they left behind. 'Why would you lie about that?' I quizzed. Imagine crying into a bereavement cake full well knowing your nan was still very much alive; she probably had a piece of her own death cake with a slice of lies for good measure. The thought made me shiver; at least it confirmed another reason why mine and Nina's friendship perished. The same couldn't be said for her nan, though, blimey. I only wanted to pick a petunia with Grandma as a relaxing day off; I wasn't planning on witnessing a weird rendition of A Christmas Carol. Except this time, it wasn't the Ghost of Christmas Past. It was the Ghost of Bullshit's Past.

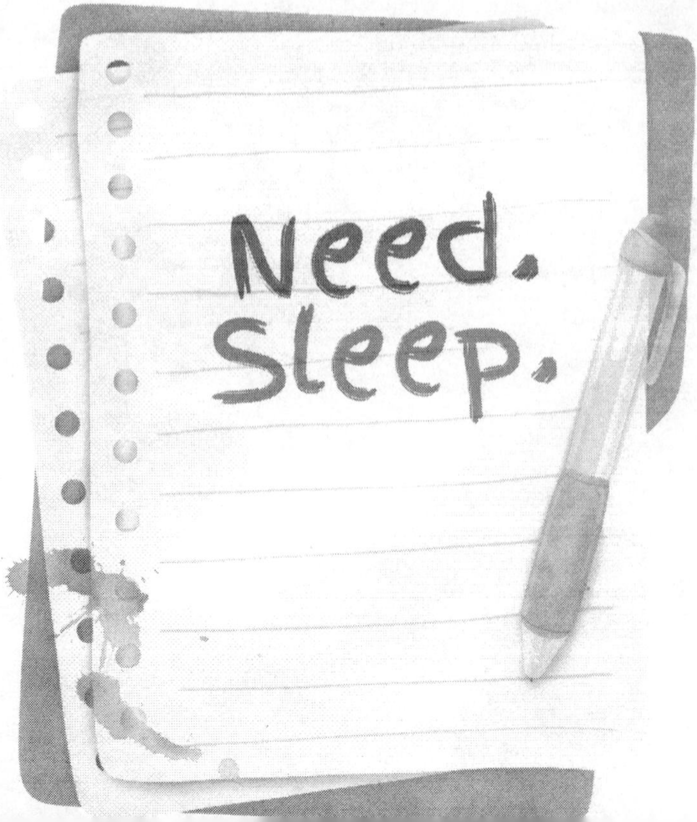
Need.
Sleep.

CHAPTER
Forty-One

THE CRUELTY LESSON: HOW NOT TO TEACH A STUDENT MIDWIFE

Following Nina's nan's surprise resurrection, I had a few more weeks of busy shifts on the unit, where I learnt a whole bunch more. After a chaotic stint in triage, I was back on Delivery Suite and paired with a midwife I hadn't met before: L, a total unknown. Naturally, I did what any anxiety-ridden student would do and gathered intel like a hormonal spy. The reviews were... confusing. 'She's lovely, you'll be absolutely fine!' One person chirped. 'Oh god,' another muttered, 'good luck.' That's the kind of contrast that sends a shiver down your spine. It wasn't just mixed messages, it was like a broken satnav. I'd have preferred a straight-up villain over this suspense thriller. Still, I clung to hope that she'd be one of the good ones. Spoiler: she wasn't.

'Hi L, I'm Meg, I'm down to work with you for the next three nights', I smiled.

'Right okay, great', she replied. I wiped a bead of sweat away with my forearm; it was a good start. Handover passed in a blur, the usual cocktail of half-heard names, unexplained abbreviations, and the low hum of fluorescent lighting doing little to calm my nerves. As we stepped into the corridor, L turned to me with an abruptness that made me flinch.

'What do you need?' she asked. I hesitated.

'Babies, ideally. My numbers are still low, I'm playing catch-up from last year,' I said, trying to sound upbeat, to show initiative. L rolled her eyes. 'There's more to midwifery than catching babies,' she muttered, just loud enough for others to hear. A couple of nearby midwives exchanged smirks, not cruel, but not exactly kind either. My stomach tightened. It was the same old feeling: say the wrong thing and the room tilts against you.

'Oh yes, of course,' I added quickly, backpedaling. 'It's just... I'm nearly at the end of second year and I've only got eight of forty of course.' L didn't reply. She simply turned and walked toward the office. I followed, unsure whether I'd just asked for support or sealed my own doom.

I sadly said goodbye to Becky, a lovely midwife on the day shift, and started typing up the handover on the computer.

'Are you not going to say hello first?' L questioned.

'I was just bashing the handover out,' I said doubting myself. I know now it did not matter the order, but at the time I felt under scrutiny before I'd even started. L didn't respond and walked towards room three. I followed her, obliged. We ended up swapping the multip for a different woman in the high dependency unit (HDU); she was a forceps birth with a two-litre post partum haemorrhage (PPH). Considering the threshold for a pph is 500 mls, it meant closer monitoring until condition stabilises for the mat ward where it is no longer one to one. I proceeded to have one of my worst shifts to date. L tore me to shreds. I felt crippling pressure to get things right, so much so, I'd get the simplest things wrong because I was so nervous. For example, I put the blood pressure cuff on backwards and the cuff started inflating like an armband. However, the vital difference I noticed was that when the same happened when I was with Joyce for example, I would crack a joke, pop it off and turn it back around (as funnily enough its not the end of the world), but I felt my bottom lip tremble when L huffed and asked me why I couldn't do the most simplest of things, in front of the family. For the first time in a long time, I felt the feeling of humiliation that I felt in my school days, and I did not miss it at all.

Although I couldn't say for sure, L seemed to enjoy knocking my confidence down piece by piece. As much as it's difficult to receive, criticism is part of life, but it's the way it's delivered. L made a conscious choice to criticise me in front of the family rather than pulling me to the side. She could have chosen kindness and spoken to me outside of the room, not making the smallest mistake seem like the biggest tragedy. I noticed she would leave me alone to care for the patient which was excellent for me, as I didn't have her presence and pressure over my shoulder. Although, she'd be laughing with her colleagues in the staff room and there would be mass silence on my entry.

'What do you want?' she asked as the laughter ceased.

'Sorry, I was wondering if you could help me out with a question, they've asked that I'm not sure of the answer, sorry,' I said nervously as I felt other eyes bore into me.

'So, what was the question?' She threw her hands out. I felt my body stiffen.

'Um just about which bloods are next to take and when, I wasn't sure because she's had her six-hour post PPH bloods, so, um, do we routinely do them again before she's out of HDU?' I asked nervously.

'What do you think?' She interlocked her fingers and her eyes remained fixed onto mine.

'Well, we have a postnatal hb* of 102, which is okay as we can give ferrous, but her U+Es* were not the best were they, so maybe a repeat of them?' I felt my cheeks flush red.

'What if she becomes symptomatic of anaemia and its reduced even further?' She said plainly. What's worst was that I was going to say about not needing another hb unless shes symptomatic. Before I got a chance to reply she hit me with another blow.

'If you'd looked at the dr review, they have written to do repeat U+Es in the morning.'

'It wasn't there when I checked,' I tried to defend myself slightly.

'You should have remembered, the doctors aren't just here for your patient, they will get around to documenting when they can.'

'Okay, brilliant, of course thanks so much, I was just checking before I gave an answer,' I said in a much kinder tone than she deserved. It was then that I realised no matter what I said, I couldn't win.

My chest became tighter and tighter as the night went on and at three am, L waltzed into the room and first thing she did was sigh.

'You've made a terrible mess of that bandage,' she announced, unwrapped it and proceeded to wrap it up in the same way. What a wanker. I only popped the bandage on to make the cannula a little more comfortable for the patient as she asked if I could put it on. I felt so stupid and small and tried so hard not to wear it on my face, but it was inevitable. I remember the patient looking at me with sympathy swimming in her eyes which was enough for me to begin to cry. I excused myself as L was in the room so she couldn't say I left anyone in any danger and made a direct route to the toilet in the main corridor away from Delivery Suite.

The room we were in was directly opposite the staff room and I noticed the other midwives chomping on a takeaway that I wasn't offered to be a part of which just added to the isolating segregation. I walked the fastest I was able out of Delivery Suite and into the corridor to the toilet. I slammed the bathroom door shut and felt my face fall. The number of times I made bee lines for that toilet in those three years, were impossible to count. It was reserved for my depression sessions as I came to call them.

So, I'd finally cracked, my chest was so tight I felt like I was going to pass out or something. The intensity saw me grab the sink to support me whilst I tried to catch my breath.

What had my life come to? That moment was simply horrendous for me; I couldn't bring myself to make any light of any of it and felt that sinking feeling of hopelessness devour me. I'd felt it drift in and out since moving to uni as I was homesick and didn't like the idea of life away from number forty-nine, I felt it when I failed the first presentation, I felt it when Sargent Sandra belittled me and my practice, I felt it more after baby Edward and now more than I was willing to admit.

The rest of the shift was pretty much the same, I couldn't believe I actually made it to sunrise to be honest. My confidence was sat in L's back pocket and sense of self-worth left was in the toilet cubicle. I felt like a shell of myself by the time eight o'clock came around, I hadn't eaten all night and couldn't regulate any of my feelings either. L handed over as admittedly, I sat blank and vacant.

'Can you come in here please before you go home?' L stated and gestured towards the little computer room. I didn't reply, only headed in on autopilot. Fatima was sat on one of the chairs, so thinking I was intruding I apologised and started backing out.

'No no, Fatima is supposed to be in here,' L said as she blocked my way out. There were only two chairs, Fatima of course took one and L sank her arse into the other. I was left to stand awkwardly. 'So,' L began, folding her arms. 'What's going on? Tonight's been a mess, hasn't it?'

'Well, I, um,' I struggled to even start a sentence.

'L has told me of what you can and mostly can't do and its simply not good enough for year two,' Fatima declared. 'Plus, we know about all that happened with Vivienne, so should you be here? Might be worth thinking about,' she said sternly. I wanted to cry but nothing happened, I felt robotic. I know that I was set up to fail before I even started the shift, they had already decided to hate me. Whether it was Vivienne, something going on within themselves, they decided to make my shift a terrible one. L stood up then and got closer to me which made me feel ridiculously uncomfortable if I didn't feel it already.

'You don't seem to retain anything either, you seem stressed at everything, do you actually retain anything?' She tapped her own head to give more meaning to the word 'retain' as if I didn't understand. Fatima sat in the background and smirked. My face was on fire, but I couldn't move or speak.

'You won't qualify, you can't even answer that,' L said and that was the last thing I remember, I didn't come out of that office until almost forty-five minutes later and I felt a shell of my previous self. I had three missed calls from Mum and a pile of messages. Instead of replying, I got in the car, turned the engine on and drove in a void until I landed on our driveway. No recollection of how I got there at all.

'Are you okay, Meg? You're back late!' Bea exclaimed as I saw her on the stairway. I couldn't answer. I stood frozen on the spot.

'Come on, we'll talk about it,' she gestured to me to go into my room. I walked as instructed and sat on my floor. It was the first time I'd felt somewhat safe all night.

'What happened? I'm worried about you,' Bea said as she lowered herself to take a seat next to me.

'I-don't-I-it-why', I stumbled over my own words and felt my breath getting quicker.

'Meg, you're safe now, you're with me,' Bea fiercely tried to reassure me and put her arms around me. 'Whatever happened, it's okay now,' she said kindly. 'Have you talked about it with your mentor, it was L, wasn't it?' She offered sensitively but upon hearing her name, I involuntarily shot up from the floor and I bolted it out of my room and into the garden. Bea was right behind me.

'I-Bea-it was her, L', I said through chest tightness.

'Whatever it is, we will sort it', she held her arms out for me, but I felt another wave of panic come over me and sat myself on the grass behind the bush so none of the other girls could see me.

'Meg, I promise you are safe, you're with me, no one else can see you.' For anyone looking on to our garden, Bea was talking to a bush and from my end I was in a ball breathing in and out of a blue glove that I had in my pocket from placement. I don't remember a lot else until my phone starting to ring.

'What the, she's found me on facebook?' I strung that sentence together just fine.

'No, stop, what?' Bea stared shocked. 'Don't you dare answer it!' Bea saw the temptation in my eyes. 'If she says one word out of line', Bea almost flexed her shoulders. She loved me fiercely and was willing to fight, always. I reluctantly pressed the green button.

'Hello,' I said in a monotonous tone whilst Bea helped me put her on speaker.

'Oh, is that Megan?' She sounded worried, a tone I'd not heard yet.

'Yes', I replied bluntly.

'Are you okay?' She asked sympathetically. She was capable after all. What on earth was going on? Had I lived a completely different night shift? 'Megan?' She continued. Bea nodded sternly at me as if to tell me to speak my truth. I guess it was my chance.

'No, I'm not actually, I think I'm broken', I stopped due to a rising pressure in my chest yet again.

'Oh god, I never meant for this to happen,' L said through a stuffy nose. Was she... crying? Why on earth was *she* crying? Had we lived the same shift? Or had she been floating through some alternate reality where undermining a student builds character?

'I had no idea what you'd really faced, you should have told me!' She exclaimed. Who on earth had she spoken with? 'Maybe we can start again?' She offered. Absolutely not.

'I don't think so, I don't think I'm coming back actually,' I said whilst my chin quivered faster than my brain could think.

'I'm still going to recommend that you shouldn't pass, but I had no idea you had no Delivery Suite in first year and when you did come to second year you had that awful event.' Why was that the biggest contradictory opinion I'd heard? Basically, I get there's a reason why you're shit now, but I still think you're shit. Did she think this was going to make up for such a horrific shift?

'I understand a bit more now, but you've got a long way to be qualified,' she reiterated. One minute she's telling me I'm shit, next thing she's alluding to me qualifying. Bea signed to me to round it up and mouthed 'this isn't helpful anymore'. She was right.

'I need to go now, I can't concentrate or regulate myself at the moment', I said through more tears.

'Well, I'll see you for tonight's shift, yes?' She questioned.

'No, probably not, I feel like I don't even know who I am,' I answered honesty, still in shock that I'm even talking to this absolute terror on the phone after twelve hours of hell.

'Please give me a chance to help you. Come back tonight, I know you can do it, I've heard you can do it,' she said too little and way too late. She lost me in handover all those hours ago.

'I really need to go, thanks for calling,' I lied through my teeth.

'Okay well, I'll see you later, try for a good sleep Megan,' she said and hung up before I hand the opportunity to reply.

'What the actual hell was that all about please?' Bea looked absolutely gobsmacked.

'I have absolutely no idea, did that just happen?' I felt genuinely confused. 'She was horrific to me Bea, I haven't even told you a thing yet', I stammered.

'She sounded bad enough there, even her trying to apologise or help still involved tearing you down!' Bea spat out in frustration. 'So, it was absolute bullshit!' She exclaimed. I laughed a little for the first time in what felt like a long time and that was because Bea wasn't a natural swearer. It took her a lot to reach that. I spent the best part of that day in a ball on Bea's bed. Thankfully she was on a day off and needed to do some work, so we had my laptop playing Below Deck and hers on her essay. I hit the lottery for friendship but lost everything when it came to hospital placement. I told Bea in fragments. I couldn't handle the full picture yet, not out loud. Not all at once.

'I need to leave, I can't do that, or Delivery Suite or X, ever again Bea, I don't actually think it's worth feeling like this,' I felt my eyebrows crease again as I cried heavier on her chest. Bea tired to persuade me to stay but understood all the reasons why I had come to the decision to stop it all. Looking back, I still don't know if L was trying to help in her own twisted way as she confused me when she called me after that shift. What I do know is that kindness teaches more than cruelty ever can.

*Hb - Haemoglobin - Essentially your iron level. Ideally, we want it to be 10.5 or 105 and above at the very least. Less than that we hit the territory of anaemia.

*U+Es – Urea and Electrolytes. This test looks at kidney function and electrolyte levels in the body. A shift in balance can cause a cascade of problems.

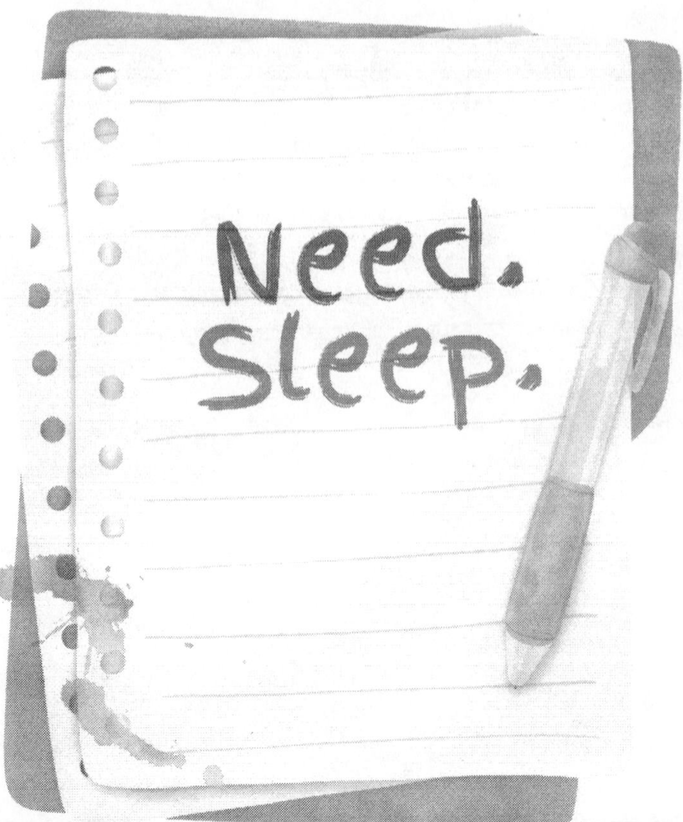
Need.
Sleep.

CHAPTER *Forty-Two*

THERE'S NO PLACE LIKE HOME

I couldn't envision myself ever returning to midwifery after that fateful day and the next few weeks were critical for me. Bea got angrier as the days passed. She saw firsthand the damage that toxic culture had done to someone who used to be so hopeful. I emailed the uni to ask for transfer from X as my limit had been exceeded that was for sure. I felt much better after that was sent as a productive action to ending the pain at least. The last thing I wanted to do was drop out as I'd leave with nothing and all of the horrible midwives would have won. I felt I'd be the biggest disappointment to my wonderful parents who always believed in me, my grandparents who always beamed when they talked about my chosen career pathway, or my wonderful teachers that put in so much extra time and hot chocolate (thanks again, Dr C), into helping me achieve what I felt I then couldn't. So, although I felt that I had nothing; what I did have was some wonderful friends and family who rallied around me to help me. I'll forever be grateful to each and every one of them.

I naively returned for a shift when everyone who loved me strongly advised me to take a bit of time out. Finally recognising that I needed to protect my vulnerable mind, I bailed out of X's Maternity Ward mid night shift. I called Mum, who answered immediately.

'I can't do it, Mum,' I instantly started crying.

'Oh Meg, come home, where are you?'

'I'm heading for the car, I just, can't, they,' I tripped over my words and began to sob.

'Can you drive home to us?' Mum asked softly.

'I think so,' I said slowly.

The drive home was odd in many ways. Firstly, the roads were eerily quiet, seen as it was 01.55 on a Sunday morning, the cars I did see were few and very far between. I had my windows cracked open and felt the force of the cold air ripple across my face as I drove toward the motherland. Just under an hour later, I arrived at forty-nine and brought my car to a stop at the back garden gates. I sat for a moment and for once my mind pressed pause, my racing thoughts frozen in limbo. I was able to hear the silence around me, and I felt a moment of peace.

I looked out at the supposedly stationary world around me, where all houses had their lights off, deep in a restful state of sleep I hoped (although half are probably battling insomnia and their racing thoughts like the majority of us).

Anyway, I stepped out of my car and into the cool air. I looked up and appreciated the great light emitting from the stars so far away and hoped for something, somewhere to guide me through the next part of my life. I turned the corner to face the front of the house and noted one room dimly lit. With that, Mum opened the door and a tired Dalmatian hopped out of the house to greet me and I burst into tears, racing thoughts on fast forward once again.

At least I was in the safest place I'd ever known, so I let it out. Mum and Dad had both waited up for me and we spent the next few hours of the morning talking everything over honestly. No sugar coating, no downplaying, a true account of events.

'So, you email the uni and explain like you did here,' Mum reiterated our formulated plan.

'If they don't help you well, I'll get involved and they'll soon buck their ideas up,' Dad supported.

'I've just been let down by literally everyone, at every stage, like that lecturer who came to support at the interview for that baby with the really poor outcome. She sat on teams with her mic and video off and didn't catch up with me afterwards either, what's the point?' I took a breath having talked about baby Edward for the first time in months. 'Then, I genuinely dragged myself into X to return to that place and then I get horrible midwives telling me its all my fault etc, ugh, yeah, it's just gone wrong at every contact since,' I started to cry once more.

'They're horrible witches Meg, seriously, you shouldn't ever be treated the way you have done and its about time that bloody place listened to you!' Mum rose a little in her chair with frustration.

'Email, wait to hear about a transfer or at least different mentors, go from there,' Dad recapped. 'And don't quit as you can do hard things and we are not going to let them win,' he said sternly.

I later retired to my room and wished I could stay in that bubble forever. Through the tears, a memory found its way through the negative storm. *For a rainy day.* I sniffed strongly as if to shoot my tears back up, for recycling. I dug around my room until I found a little folded post it note.

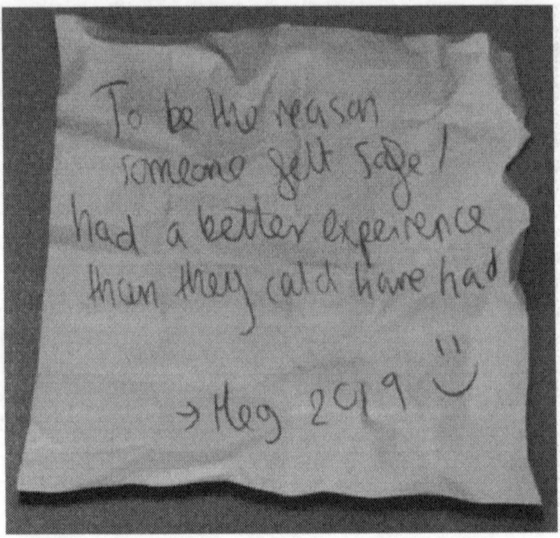

I realised I had been shown the opposite some disgustingly behaved mentors. I cried until I couldn't cry anymore.

CHAPTER

Forty-Three

BREATHING THROUGH BLUE LATEX

After some restorative time with my parents, siblings and the dog, I had just arrived back at our student house and received an email from uni to say they had rejected my plea for a change of trust, so it was X or nothing. Devastated was an understatement. After all of the frank bullying, panic attacks and poor clinical outcomes, I'd panic as soon as I'd step over the hospital's threshold and hated X more than I ever had. Although, I felt some budding self loathing that slowly edged its way into my life; I felt embarrassed and useless to all of the midwives with no idea of my place in the world. At least I knew where I didn't fit in, nevertheless, that isolation left me in an empty void of sadness and uncertainty.

As anticipated, my mental health deteriorated and a few weeks down the line I couldn't even string a sentence together as the ongoing anxiety trapped me under its spell. I spent hours having prolonged panic attacks on the floor, for so long once, I didn't eat or drink for the best part of the day. One of the girls used to bring me blue gloves home from the hospital she went to, and I used them like a paper bag to try and regulate something. I remember Bea finally convinced me to go to the GP and the doctor was quite surprised that I hadn't presented before it had hit the severity it had. Even so, they fixed me up with a prescription of anti-anxiety and anti-depressant medication, which was impressive for someone who was quite anti-everything at the time. I commenced counselling with a psychotherapist who specialised in EMDR (eye movement desensitisation and reprocessing) and it was life changing. It wasn't instant. But little by little, the EMDR sessions started to untangle the horror in my head. I learned to say: what happened to that baby was awful, but it wasn't my fault. I said it out loud one day in therapy and burst into tears. But I didn't feel broken anymore. Just human.

CHAPTER
Forty-Four

MIDWIVES, NOT MONSTERS

Mum said my light slowly came back to me, one warm day, one full night's sleep, one belly laugh at a time. After months of recovery, the end of June brought warmer weather, and with it, a fragile feeling of readiness. I decided to give Delivery Suite one last shot. This time, with different mentors. I was thankful to the uni and hospital for recognising that was what I needed in order to return. Even still, the anxiety was overpowering. I just kept reminding myself: this was temporary. One day, I'd wash my hands of the place, for good. It was a little like my GCSE years again; I had the strongest motivation to pass and get my one-way ticket out of there and toward better things.

I wasn't magically healed, but this time I was paired with Millie and Caz, two mentors who reminded me what midwifery could look like when empathy leads. I felt nothing but terror when I stepped back over the clinical threshold, memories flooded back like that flash flood of 2013. Millie and Caz saw it in me, and they treated me with compassion, kindness and gave me the space to be comfortable and progress.

Like true outstanding mentors. We had many births of many modes, haemorrhages, general anaesthetics, PET, sepsis, the lot. I learnt so much and felt like I could actually beat this thing, finally. Bea remained my rock throughout it all and we spent many days off doing mindful or fun things as a reminder that life could be good and there was more to life than work. Although, I did lose my apple watch when we did an aqua park course in the middle of a lake in the wilderness. I remember asking the guy if there was any way we could get it back and he told me it was a categorical no and that mine was probably the hundredth one lost to the lake by now.

So, if you're ever struggling and need a small fortune, it lies at the bottom of the lake in the Cotswolds, certainly not at X hospital.

My favourite discovery was not my watch, but that Millie and Caz saw no issues at all with my practice, and I had passed my second year, giving rise to a hopeful and restorative summer. I was so grateful, I remember how dreamy it felt to just sit in the garden and absorb the world around me. I related a little when a few patients I looked after over the last two years mentioned mum's guilt. However, mine was with my academics, like revision guilt. It became a huge and realistic phenomenon, but after receiving the jolly news of passing onto level three, I could relish a few weeks off for what they were, unstructured and free. I intentionally spent lots of time with the dog, although the last time I took him on a walk, he retched and threw up his stomach contents mid-walk. It took him a few minutes to recover, but all was well in the end. The builders downed tools and stared straight at me. From their angle, the dog was invisible. I considered shouting 'It wasn't me!' but just nodded like a woman who'd made peace with vomiting in public. Bloody brilliant.

PART 3

YEAR 3

CHAPTER

Forty-Five

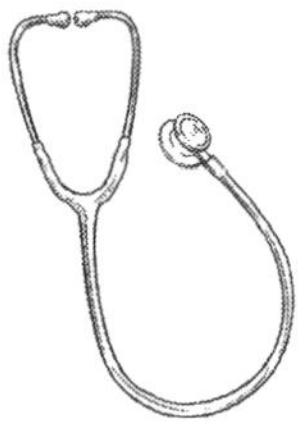

FULL CIRCLES

September 2021. Back to Worcester, for the beginning of the end of my degree. Sitting in the familiar groove of the lecture hall seat, I turned to Bea and looked up at the screen: *Welcome to your third and final year.* A lot had happened since I was last in this room, wide-eyed at an open day, flipping a fifty pence piece like it was my academic advisor.

'Eleven dropouts,' Lynsey said, pausing for effect like she was announcing who wouldn't be returning to the board-room on The Apprentice. 'Twenty-two remain.' Exactly as she'd predicted two years ago.

'It's a time to reflect, be proud of what you've achieved, and how far you've come,' Annie beamed at the survivors, as we were made to feel.

'Here we go again,' Bea smiled at me. I nodded. I'd met some incredible people as friends, mentors, and lecturers, who I know changed my life for the better. I learnt that a drop of kindness goes a long way toward blossoming new possibilities and building imperative, positive self-esteem. But I'd also met people who made me question how anyone could be so persistently cruel. Part of me wondered what had happened to them.

Another part just wanted them out of my brain, permanently. The damage they'd done, the depression, the embarrassment, the weight of feeling worthless, was real. There's no excuse for that. We all have off days; I've definitely had mine. But there's a difference between being occasionally short and being consistently awful. For those people: get help. Stop punishing the rest of us for your demons.

'This year will be the toughest', Lynsey warned as I zoned back into her voice. 'You'll need to rely on your friends and family!' She went on to say. Bea and I exchanged a look to wonder how it would get much worse than it already had. But the beauty in it was that I didn't feel half as anxious as I would have without her there with me. We complimented each other beautifully, and whatever was to come, a major pivotal point in my life was that I had managed to find someone so wonderful throughout it all. Cheers to us, Mecca.

Lynsey and Annie carried on and discussed the course layout for year three and man it was intense. This week's itinerary was to prepare to teach second-year neonatal resuscitation. Like sorry? I have a) not been on placement for months and b) have only ever scribed during such an emergency. I thought second year was bad. I felt all the pride and inspiration I felt at the start of the evaporate by the time I clambered into my bed at nine o'clock that evening. I lay flat on my back with the third-year itinerary on my chest, staring at the ceiling like it might beam down the answers. Welcome to your third and final year, I thought, right before I passed out into the sweet escape of unconsciousness.

CHAPTER
Forty-Six

LONE BIRTH

We did end up teaching the second-year students neonatal resuscitation, did group presentations on contemporary midwifery practice and started an essay on critiquing a research paper. By the time October came around, my brain was stretched to every corner, and we were released back out to placement. Yet again I was placed in X. First up, community and thankfully it meant the return of the one, the only, Joyce. I'd missed our adventures, and she welcomed me back with open arms which felt like a rare and wonderful thing. We had a lovely four weeks where we managed to avoid hills, sheep and shit. I also managed to get all of my community proficiencies signed off for the third year and Joyce even wrote me a card to say how proud she was of how far I'd come. I couldn't have felt happier. Big up Joyce, always.

November I was headed back for Delivery Suite. Overly focused on the long night ahead of me as a third year now and the dreaded expectations, I didn't notice the peace that the evening sky brought to the hospital I'd grown to resent. Instead, I was hurrying down the narrow path towards the staff entrance with a flurry of thoughts whisking through my head. What would tonight be like? Would bitch-face Lottie be there? Sergeant Sandra? I was always more hyper-focused on the people as they were half the battle for me. Plus, with a small unit, everyone knew everyone. Advantageous if your face fit, but if it didn't, boy did you know about it.

Devoured in my thoughts, I had arrived at Delivery Suite's doors before I even registered, I had. I pressed the worn-out buzzer attached to the side of the doors hard and waited. I never got given an access pass, the matron said students weren't a priority for passes, especially if they might drop out anyway. Charming. Even so, three years into working there they *still* didn't view me as eligible for one when I emailed in September. That was the thing, I didn't matter, and three long years had all the proof I needed...

'Hello, midwife speaking,' came a muffled voice through the radio. Pretty sure it was Victoria.

'Hello, it's Meg,' I said quite happily considering the dread I felt.

'Meg who?' A cold voice replied instantly.

'Meg, student midwife?' I replied flatly. Third and final year and she still didn't give a toss as to who I was. There was a long sigh through the radio and the doors clicked open. I opened them with regret and headed down the Main Street of Delivery Suite. With still only five delivery rooms, it made X one of the smallest maternity units in the country. Trying to get forty unassisted vaginal births was difficult at the best of times let alone in a unit that a lot of the time had one birth a century.

I smiled at Kate as I scurried along the corridor, she was one of the nice midwives that I had a few good shifts with before, but I quickly realised she was on the day shift which only made my smile fade quicker as I headed for the changing rooms. As we all know, when the supportive midwives were there, I felt as though I could conquer the world in one night while the rest of the town slept. However, on the contrary, those that made life very difficult for students were shifts that made you feel as though that world was chewing you up and spitting you back out, into an eternity of isolation.

'Ahh, Meg, how are you chick?' A voice said beaming from behind me. I swivelled around knowing exactly who it was and let out a sigh of relief.

'Jess! Lovely to see you, you on the night? How are things?' I said gladly.

'Good, good my lovely, and yes, I am. On the night it seems, in for a quiet one, one in labour. Well not for you I guess Meg, you need those births, how many is it to go now?' Jess said it all in what seemed like one breath as she wiped her blonde bangs away from her eyes.

'Oh um, yeah, I have twenty-eight at the mo, so twelve to go!' I took a breath. 'Nearly there, I tell myself they'll come eventually!' I said optimistically.

'Most end in theatre these days though, don't you think Edith?' She turned my attention to a midwife who was sitting still on a chair in the corner of the changing room. Not *Edith.* A particularly brutal band seven midwife in charge often will show her authority by shouting orders at anyone with an ID badge. She once barked at a man in green scrubs waiting outside of the drugs cupboard demanding him to 'get on with his work and not just stand there blocking her cupboard.' Turned out he was from the pharmacy waiting for the midwife to come out of said cupboard to sign the form to say she had put out control drugs safely into the right place. Dickhead. Many people thought her attitude was just 'old school'. I often wondered if 'just old school' was code for plain incivility, rudeness and general bad feeling. Something to have a think about. Anyway, why did it have to be Edith? I buried her face into my tunic and hoped I could have stayed like that for the rest of the night.

Time doesn't wait for anyone though, and as on every other shift, I meandered may way to the tiny little room for handover. It was a Sunday night shift and as Jess had correctly said, one woman in labour tonight, so naturally, she was assigned to us. Jess flashed an encouraging smile towards me, and I knew her brain was ticking away on something.

'Solo?' I said worriedly. 'Are you mad?' I said laughing.

'I'm deadly serious Meg; you can do this! I trust you,' Jess replied.

'Haha, Jess, I'm glad you bloody do,' I felt the panic rise a little. I hadn't been there for months.

'Come off it, you do. I'll obviously be involved,' Jess reassured me. 'She's low-risk Meg, induction for postdates,' I could feel my brain ticking, trying to figure out what I needed to do and why. Jess could see the cogs turning.

'Come onnnn, you make the plan, inform me, I tweak it, if necessary,' Jess encouraged me.

'When you're in there, press the call bell if you need any help, yeah?' Jess adds cooly.

'You make it sound so easy!' I said still laughing yet doubting my abilities. Nothing new there.

'I'll be outside, just shout if you need any help Meg,' Jess says after introducing herself to the woman and her partner and gaining consent for me to be her lead with Jess moments away.

'I'm shouting,' I said both quietly and nervously. Jess laughed back and shook her head.

'Get in there gal!' Jess said giving me a rather hard pat on the back between my shoulder blades. I stretched my arms out in front of me, shook my head and wiggled my toes. You're going to do this, Meg. Positive affirmation, let's go. A friend once told me that she looks in the mirror every morning and tells herself she can do it, and she always goes on to do it.

Positive affirmation. I envisioned myself desperately screaming at the mirror in the dirty utility (all sorts happen in that place) and begging it for a little guidance. I quickly brought myself back to the real world, pushed my fears to one side and knocked on the door. Peering around the corner of the curtain, I found a lady reading a book on the delivery bed with her glasses perched on the bridge of her nose. The birth wasn't imminent. Thank fuck. I remember staring at her in relief. Realising that I should probably introduce myself rather than looking as though I was trying to find a brain cell to count on for conversation, I made my introductions.

Abbie was cool, calm and collected. She told me she didn't really want induction and wasn't keen on any further intervention at that point. She felt like her body had got it going on. I liked her certainty and confidence in her body. The only issue with that was if it did go tits up. We talked about it and decided to cross that bridge if it came to it. The next step was putting it all in writing; handover of care, six hundred different risk assessments and the care plan moving forward. I eventually found time to ask Abbie my usual spiel of 'do you know what you're having? I bet you're excited to meet baby now; do you have any names in the air?' The answer tonight was a little boy, however, unsure of her name.

'Ooo how exciting!' I chirped. My answer was the same as it always was, with always the same feigned delight. Abbie was receptive to it, and we hit it off well.

Time went on and Abbie seemed to be getting more uncomfortable. She declined to monitor for the next hour whilst she was in the bath and didn't want to be disturbed. Fair play. I chatted to her partner, Ross about the restaurant they own, when I heard the obstetricians practically knocking the door down. About time. Ward round, at about a night shift too late that night. Usually, it's because something's going drastically wrong somewhere, but I had the only occupied room. Anyway, I sprinted across the room to greet them for the handover.

I communicated the situation to the doctors whereby they all just stared as I nervously spat the info out like a robot. They asked if she'd had her waters broken yet as per the plan.

'No, we've discussed why we recommend it, and she declined, she feels as though her body is doing what it needs to do off the back of the propess*, and to be fair she's contracting, but not regularly at present time,' I answered honestly.

'Well, that's just ridiculous,' one of the doctors exclaims in response. The other doctors laughed alongside and whispered things that they wouldn't say in front of the woman like 'get your scrubs on,' or 'asking for a section.' Not all doctors had those outlooks, often far from it. But equally, a lot have been so caught up in the disasters they've seen, it understandably becomes harder to see the potential for normal physiology in a modern world of pathology.

'Well, she wants the minimal amount of intervention, so unless anything crops up as unsafe, she's happy to ride the waves,' I tried to convince their medicalised minds.

'She's riding the waves to an exclusive emergency delivery in theatre,' the consultant chipped in. Bastards.

A few hours later, I was due to offer Abbie an examination. I'd checked with Jess, and she was in agreement. Thankfully. Jess followed me into the room for that part but as soon as we walked across the threshold Abbie was in all fours swaying on the bed.

'Meg, I feel so much pressure,' she announced calmly.

'Fantastic! That's always something we love to hear,' I replied concealing the nerves and excitement that started to bubble from within. Jess and I discussed the plan from here. Abbie's behaviour was starting to change. She was contracting regularly now too. With all of this in consideration, Jess and I were more than happy to skip the examination, and Abbie wanted the minimal amount anyway. Jess left me to it again and I was faced with the task of filling the pool. It was an inflatable one but had space for the taps to sit on the edge. I pushed the taps to full speed and reassured Abbie it shouldn't be too long. She was making different noises and asking her husband to politely fuck off every time he touched her back even though that's what he had been doing to help up until now. A trusty sign of transition. Birth wouldn't be far away now, but the pool was.

About half an hour moved quickly and surprisingly baby wasn't as close as we thought. I was worried about filling the pool in time, but now I beat myself up for overfilling it. I was so focused on Abbie's behaviour, and monitoring the baby, that my last priority was the pool. The water gleamed precariously at the edge of the tub. Abbie had what was deemed a 'normal' BMI even though BMI was based on white men of a certain age (another story for another time), if she were to get in now, she'd send a tidal wave right the way through Delivery Suite and clear up the dead wood along the way. I had intrusive visions about more than just crumpled infrastructure, wiping Edith off her perch? Maybe it wasn't the worst idea.

Thinking about it, it's a shame she didn't have a bigger BMI or I couldn't dive bomb in there, as the thought of sending a tsunami through to the front desk, capable of finishing Edith off for good was really appealing, especially as I had another nine hours of sharing the same building as her. I could just see it, I'd actually wave her off to her slightly earlier retirement. I chuckled to myself until I went to reach for the plug but couldn't see it. I couldn't see anything at all. What? I swung my head around one side of the pool and the other, no connections, no tubes. What is the actual? This goes to show how few water births I'd been involved in. The 'low risk' was far rarer than their opposition. Still, where was the fucking plug?

I frantically assessed my surroundings thinking how the bloody hell I was going to empty this a little. Dangerously, Abbie was on all fours now and intermittently mooing. A multip mooing and telling me she can't do it anymore? The baby was imminent. Shit. What was I going to say when she asked if the pool was ready again? Oh, hold on, I just need to figure out how to get water out of a free-standing inflatable pool. Surely it couldn't be that hard. I quickly popped out of the room to find Jess but instead was faced with Edith. UGH.

'What have you done now?' She paused her conversation with another midwife to ask me.

'Nothing, have you seen Jess?' I asked trying to conceal the rising urgency.

'She's gone to help someone in another room at the moment. Can we answer your questions?' She asked with a smirk on her face, and I knew she only offered so she could mock me.

'No thankyou, just to inform her that I think our lady is cracking on is all,' I said in a tone much nicer than intended.

'Well, you shouldn't be out here then should you,' she said with a nasty undertone. I couldn't win.

I quickly went back into my room to find Abbie in the same position and occasionally bearing down for a moment or so. Bollocks. Right stand-alone pool, no plug, no connection to anything. How on earth do you empty this thing, seriously, I couldn't think of a rational explanation. I couldn't ask Edith, she would roast me then fire me from a job I do for free anyway. So, I had to improvise. I eyed up a mug on the side of the table and a sink in touching distance of the pool. Abbie and Ross were still facing away from me, so I took my chance and grabbed the mug dunked it in the depths and mug by mug, threw the water in the sink.

I was on hyper speed, chucking water at the sink and splashing myself in the meantime. I listened to the baby's heart rate frequently still, only to return to the pool in between. I carried on as both parents didn't notice me and wondered worriedly where on earth Jess was. Finally, after breaking a sweat, the pool was at least enterable.

'Abbie, we're ready for you,' I said proudly and slightly out of breath.

'Thankyou, Meg, appreciate your effort,' she said with utter relief. Appreciate your effort? I know all mums have eyes on the back of their heads, but surely not! Regardless, Ross and I helped her off the bed, however, after a few steps she stopped to give an almighty push down.

'He's coming!' Abbie exclaimed then quite literally threw herself in the pool. Thought I'd have to dive in after her, she was only little. I wondered where champion diving Tommy was at in that moment but was quickly distracted when Abbie pushed again. I pressed the call bell in the room for someone to come into a) get me a qualified midwife and b) get me a second qualified midwife as I could see the top of the baby's head now. Nobody came. But I also couldn't leave as coaching someone through this part was crucial for so many reasons. Thankfully baby's heart rate remained the same so no concerns at present, however, I CALLED THE BLOODY MIDWIFE, where was she?

Abbie's body was moving too quick for any of us and baby's head made an appearance with the next contraction. My call bell was still going. I brought the towel down from my shoulder and on the next contraction, baby made an appearance, and finally, so did Jess!

'Bloody heck Meg,' she laughed, 'that was quick!' She declared the obvious to us all.

'Congratulations Abbie!' I said as I rubbed her little boy, and he started to cry. I felt like doing the same, to be honest. I shouldn't have been on my own in there. Although it felt kind of brilliant.

I felt a massive amount of pride and was so glad Jess had literally chucked me in at the deep end and thought things were finally coming together until one of our Maternity Support Workers (MCAs) came in to empty the pool. She brought a huge contraption on wheels with her. I pretended to faff around with something so I could observe this. She pulled out a massive tube, shoved one side in the pool and the other in the toilet and flicked the switch. The contraption sucked all of the water and debris out of the pool and into the toilet, in approximately ten minutes. Imagine whipping that out whilst someone is mid labouring, about to push their baby out and I'm there with big machinery which sounds like I'm drilling into the pool. Not quite the serene birthing experience. Thankfully and most importantly, both parents didn't seem to notice or be affected by my pool emptying skills and in fact, they dropped a card in a week later, gifting me a free pass to have a meal at their restaurant. Result!

* A propess is a prostaglandin we use to kick-start induction. Every trust has its favourite trick, but ours was the trusty propess. Picture a tiny tampon parked at the cervix, quietly dripping out hormones for twenty-four hours straight. The midwifery version of subtle persuasion. Basically, the baby's first eviction notice.

CHAPTER
Forty-Seven

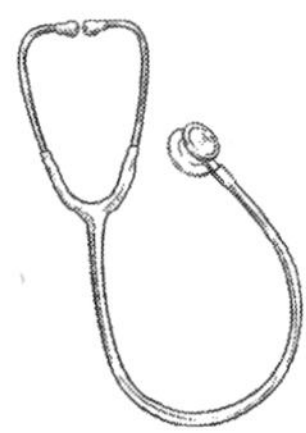

MATERNITY WARD: WHERE PLANS GO TO DIE AND CTGS MULTIPLY

X's Maternity ward: both antenatal and postnatal women are together. The antenatal side always seemed more complex where people warded were at high risk for plenty of different reasons; pv bleeding, threatened pre-term labour, hypertension, inductions, infections, it was a frenzy of complications. Keeping up with every woman's story and situation was also quite a task. Although we had online maternity notes, I've yet to find a midwife who doesn't use paper for some reason or another. Most handovers received involve folding a piece of A4 into quarters and assigning a woman a square each. On one of my antenatal days my mentor, Aimee had six antenatal women in for all sorts. I crammed their situations down and Aimee taught me how to organise my time on the ward with the following timetable, a timetable I still use now:

TABLE KEY:

- SBAR - Handover of care - Situation, Background, Assessment, Recommendation.
- Reg - Registrar, specialist doctor
- CTG - Cardiotocograph
- A1-4 - A bay, with the numbers representing the patient occupying it.
- R1-2 - Rooms 1+2.
- VTE - Venous Thromboembolism
- Obs - Observations - pulse, temp, SATS, blood pressure, FHR.

8.00	9.00	10.00	11.00
SBAR A1 A2 A3 A4 R1 R2 For anytime of day: Urine dip + VTE assessments A1 A2 A3 A4 R1 R2	Antibiotic A1 Review A1 A3 A4 Blood sugar R1 CTG R1	Obs A1 A2 A3 A4 R1 R2 Anticoagulant R1 CTG A4	CTG A1 Labetalol A4 Reassess A2
12.00	13.00	14.00	15.00
Bloods A3		Obs A1 A2 A3 A4 R1 R2 Blood sugar R1	A3 CTG, take propess out, reassess +/- prostin*
16.00	17.00	18.00	19.00
Steroids R2 CTG A4	CTG and take Cooke's Balloon* out A2 Labetalol A4 Antibiotic A1	Obs A1 A2 A3 A4 R1 R2	

At least it made the day seem more manageable which it was until someone had complications and shit hit the fan whereby the rest of the tasks became late, reshuffled or changed entirely. The revised timetable of reality went a bit like this:

8.00	9.00	10.00	11.00
SBAR A1 ✓ A2 ✓ A3 ✓ A4 ✓ R1 ✓ R2 ✓ For anytime of day: Urine dip + VTE assessments A1 ✓ ✓ A2 ✓ ✓ A3 ✓ ✓ A4 ✓ ✓ R1 ✓ ✓ R2 ✓ ✓	Antibiotic A1 ✓ Review A1 ✓ A3 ✓ A4 Blood sugar R1 ✓ CTG R1 ✓	Obs A1 ✓ A2 ✓ A3 ✓ A4 ✓ R1 R2 CTG A4 ✓ Anticoagulant R1 ✓ Send A1 drugs chest to pharmacy ✓	~~CTG A1~~ Labetalol A4 ✓ CTG A4 ✓ Obs A4 ✓ R1 ✓ R2 ✓ Discharge A1
12.00	**13.00**	**14.00**	**15.00**
~~Bloods A3~~ CTG A1 ✓ Discharge A1 ✓ ~~Repeat A4 BP~~	Bloods A3 ✓ SBAR for new A1 ✓ Repeat A4 Bp ✓ Bleeding reg A4 ✓ Nifedipine A4 ✓	Obs A1 ✓ A2 ✓ A3 ✓ A4 ✓ R1 ✓ R2 ✓ Blood sugar R1 ✓ CTG R1 ✓ Metformin/Insulin? R1 ✓	A3 CTG, take propess out, reassess +/- Prostin ✓ ✓ ✓ ~~Steroids R2~~ Blood sugar R1 ✓
16.00	**17.00**	**18.00**	**19.00**
Reg review A3 ✓ Cannula A3 ✓ Bloods A3 ✓ CTG review A3 ✓ ~~CTG A4~~	Reassess A3 ✓ ~~CTG and take Cooke's Balloon out A2~~ Labetalol A4 ✓ ~~Antibiotic A1~~	Obs ~~A1~~ ~~A2~~ ~~A3~~ A4 ✓ ~~R1~~ R2 ✓ SBAR new A3 ✓	Steroids R2 ✓ Obs A1 ✓ A2 ✓ A3 ✓ R1 ✓

For context;

- A1 was confirmed to have flu and doctors prescribed her oral antibiotics, so she went home to carry on having flu there instead.
- A2's Cooke's balloon fell out at 11.00 so we reassessed her then and she was a good three centimetres

and the look on her face resembled that of a child on Christmas Day. I felt second hand happiness for her.

- A3's cervix wasn't favourable once we took the first induction agent out but when we put the Prostin in, her baby didn't respond well, so she spent two hours on the CTG whilst we attempted to fix things with IVs (intra venous infusions), shuffling her into different positions, she even tried a glass of milk which she was convinced was the reason her baby wasn't happy because 'he gets upset when she doesn't drink it'. However, on this occasion, I think it was the prostaglandin as unfortunately the milk did nothing. She had to go to Delivery Suite in the end for close monitoring/1:1 care that we couldn't facilitate.
- A4 had high bloody pressure at 10.00 in stroke territory at 181/115, gave her medication asap. We commenced and completed a thankfully normal CTG. However, when I went in to repeat her blood pressure at 12.00 to hopefully see an improvement after medication she wasn't there! She wandered back at about half one smelling of 'the devil's lettuce' as one midwife described but at least she had a lower blood pressure. Was it the medication or the lord's green leaves? Either way, both seemed quite ineffective, it seemed to take an age to get her blood pressure down to what we deemed as normal, but we finally got there at about half past three.
- New A1 was a lady in for a CTG three times a day due to reporting absent fetal movements and was

naturally scared out of her mind so I spent about forty minutes in her space alone. I hope it helped.

- Room 1 was okay until she spiked her blood sugar at 14.00 at ten point five. I told her to try and go for a walk around the ward, gave her her medication and we would recheck it shortly. I went in to repeat it an hour later and she was necking a bottle of full-fat coke. An excellent choice for taste but not so much for her diabetes. Thankfully the threat of having a sliding scale which involved multiple cannulas, a continuous CTG and hourly blood sugar monitoring sunk in, so she binned the coke and took her adjusted dose of meds as per the doctor's plan.
- Room 2 was fuming that we didn't give her steroids on time. In fairness, they were due at 15.00 but we ended up giving them to her at 19.00 due to the above. The ward involved picking your battles and priority based on safety had to come first as you simply cannot be everywhere.

Apparently, this was one of the good days for the mat ward although I couldn't remember whose vagina belonged to who at one point...

* Prostin is another prostaglandin: basically, propess' slightly less glamorous sibling.

* Cooke's balloon, or CRB, is one of maternity's more genius ideas. Basically, we thread a catheter through the vagina into the cervix, then inflate balloons on either side. Like sticking a double-ended lilo through a letter-

box. One balloon hangs out in the uterus, keeping baby company, and the other stays in the vagina for support. We pump up to eighty mls of water into them. Google it - it looks harmless enough until you picture it wedged inside a cervix barely a centimetre open. That's when you start crossing your legs in sympathy.

CHAPTER
Forty-Eight

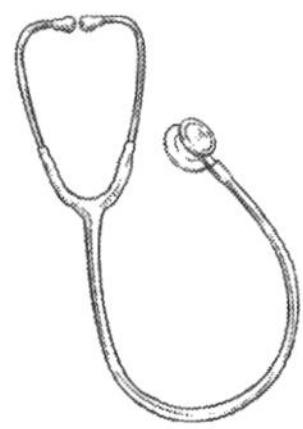

AN UNUSUAL REQUEST

The ward got a little easier as I found my way to an effective routine. However, antenatal care was very different to postnatal care and my mind had a hard time adjusting, especially if we fleeted between the two. What I loved most about ward work, though, was the people. Every room held a different family, each with its own dynamics, dramas, and quirks. Whereas on Delivery Suite, it was all of your time and energy on one person, one family, so if they were a vibe, awesome, if not, it became a little uneasy from time to time. As with everything, the different areas of midwifery had their pros and cons.

One of my favourite memories from my time on the ward was my first experience of answering a toilet call bell.

I was making my way calmly there but all of a sudden, a flurry of midwives flew past me towards the source. Looking frantically over my shoulders and realising the potential urgency, I picked up my feet and scurried after the swarm of blue. When we arrived, one midwife, Amy was rapping on the door and asking if everything was okay. No response. Another midwife searched the bay to find out who it was, but strangely, all the women were in their beds. Almost immediately, a collective decision was made to unlock the door in case there was someone unconscious behind the door and needed immediate help. I then regretted moving so casually to begin with. Sian, one of our MCAs twisted the lock and opened the door to reveal a small child sitting on the toilet with his pants to his ankles.

'Can you wipe my bum please?' He asked plainly. The tension collapsed like he'd taken the last piece out of a Jenga tower. I couldn't help but smile to myself after the adrenaline of a potential emergency dissipated. The poor guy just wanted a hand. He pointed to one of the midwives, Grace who was so furious so located his parents and sent his dad in to sort him out in the end.

'Everything okay?' The in-charge midwife had arrived now.

'Stand down, no emergency,' Grace announced seriously.

'What was it?' Another midwife at the desk asked.

'A child needing us to wipe his ass,' she said in a furious whisper.

'He must've slipped in while visiting his mum or sibling...'

The receiving midwife scuffed a little laughter as Grace stormed down the corridor to get on with her work. Brilliant. Midwifery teaches you to expect the unexpected, but sometimes, the unexpected just wants a clean bum.

CHAPTER *Forty-Nine*

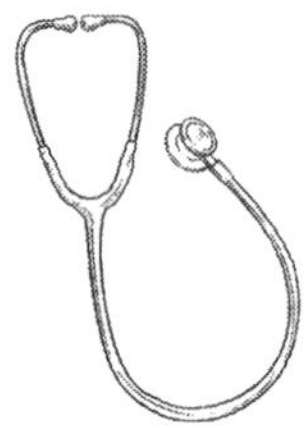

DENTISTRY OR MIDWIFERY?

On a drizzly Monday morning, I was helping care for a patient called Sandy, who was quite a serious person and I found my attempts of having a laugh with her weren't reciprocated. She looked at me blankly as I laughed at my own jokes to fill the silence. I turned the humour off and stuck to what I was being paid for in the end (or would be paid for eventually). So, Sandy was having her first baby, sitting comfortably with an effective epidural on board and the baby's head had descended well after a lot of pushing. However, it had been an hour and a half of pushing, and the baby hadn't decided to make its appearance yet. My mentor, Diane gave me the eyes of 'it's going to be a doctor job in a minute' as she was filling in the relevant paperwork. Classic.

So, I stepped up the energy and tried my best to encourage her to get this child out before the doctor needed to get involved.

'You can do it, Sandy, really you can!' I said as she resisted the next contraction.

'I can't Meg, I'm too tired,' she sighed as the contraction faded. To be fair she looked knackered, her brows were glistening with little beads of sweat, and her face looked a couple shades paler than it did earlier.

'I know it's easy for me to say but you can do this, you're doing so well!' I coached as the next contraction came along.'Push, that's it,' I continued, however, after a few seconds of pushing she consciously stopped herself and looked to be resisting it entirely.

'Do you still feel it there?' I said as I palpated her abdomen. Rock solid. 'It's still there Sandy, come on let's use it, you're so close now!' My words fell on deaf ears and no matter what I said she kept stopping herself after a few seconds.

Eventually, she said she needed not to push because it was making her feel really nauseous. I ran out of the room and flew around Delivery Suite trying and get hold of anything to help get rid of the nausea.

'I need an anti-sickness concoction people!' I said to two midwives who were staring at me as I was sprinkling peppermint oil onto a taper.

'You'll need a hell of a lot more than that if you want this baby Meg,' Diane said as she exited the room herself. 'I don't know how much more we can explain to her,' she said hopelessly whilst leaning against the cupboard. I nodded somewhat in agreement and headed back into the room.

'Have a sniff of this?' I said happily as I gave her the taper. Diane came in and supervised me as I gave her an antiemetic injection too, but she left immediately afterwards. Thanks, Diane. Meanwhile, Sandy reported feeling better, however, as Diane predicted, the situation remained the same. Contraction, push for a few moments and stop. At that moment, Sandy gagged loudly as her body took over and was involuntary pushing. I rubbed her back with my right hand and held a vomit bowl in front of her with my left.

'Better out than in,' I said as she was renching away, 'you'll probably feel the world of good once it's out,' I tried to reassure her. She looked up at me unconvinced. A moment of silence passed. This was followed by another almighty contraction with a side order of encouragement from me. Sandy pushed past her few-second limit, and I felt like a proud Mum watching her achieve her personal best. I was rooting for her so much I was pushing myself. But then she gave an almighty retch. And another. Then, like a busted garden hose, green liquid shot across the room.

Fair play, both the speed of exit and the amount were quite impressive. Before Sandy could take a breath, round two came for her and saw another shade of green, projectile vomit leave her system. I actively jumped out of the way of that one as it was travelling fast. No wonder the poor woman didn't want to push. Then I had to take a double take, but I was sure I saw something else fly amongst the third stream of vomit. It looked white and angular. My stomach dropped. Was that a *tooth?* Surely not. Nevertheless, I sprung forward and set out in the wilderness of sick to retrieve it. I picked it up before even thinking and soon Realised her tooth were teeth and her teeth were actually a whole rack of them.

'*Dentures?*' I whispered to myself in shock and turned back to face Sandy.

'Can I have my teeth back please,' she muffled as she stared at her top set of teeth cupped in my left hand.

'Gosh, bless you, I'm so sorry,' I blurted out, embarrassed. What was I sorry for? I didn't rip them out, or at least not physically. But I did encourage her to push so hard she lost her teeth...

'Right let me just,' I said as I stepped over the sick to get to the sink. I put her teeth on the side. 'You guys stay just there, and I'll get back to you in a moment,' I said to her molars as if they were a group of kids that could abscond if I didn't keep an eye. Maybe they would? Distracting myself from walking teeth, I mopped up the vomit and gave Sandy a clean gown to rid her of the smell. I wiped my forehead with my forearm as I carried the last of it to the bin.

'Back to you,' I casually addressed the teeth whilst I popped a fresh pair of gloves on. I picked them up and started to scrub this patient's teeth clean. At that moment I questioned all of my life choices thus far. I had a woman's teeth in my hands whilst she was sat there with only her bottom row in situ. She didn't find any of it funny either, which made me want to laugh more and I ended up talking to them more than her. It was bonkers. My thoughts were interrupted by a knock at the door and Diane emerged.

'So we just have the doctors coming in to see you as we've been pushing for some time,' Diane said as entered the room accompanied by the shift's obstetric registrar, Helen.

'Hi Sandy, my name's Helen and I am the obstetric registrar on shift today,' she gave a warm smile which always shone from behind her eyes. 'I've come in to chat to you about how long we've been pushing for and see what's next to allow for your baby to be born safely,' Helen said with a calming voice. She went on to explain the risks of a prolonged second stage, the CTG and options from here. Whilst she was doing so, I decided to continue subtly scrubbing so Sandy could have the reunion asap. Diane side-eyed me and double took as she watched me clean Sandy's teeth.

'What on *earth* are you doing Meg?' She whispered, her face contorted with confusion

'Don't ask,' I pursed my lips and shook my head trying to shake off the embarrassment.

'Are they *teeth?*' She smirked.

'Fifteen of the beauties,' I whispered back trying to be quiet as Helen was still discussing theatre with Sandy. Diane pointed at Sandy as if to ask me if they were her teeth. I felt my eyebrows rise as I nodded my head fiercely in confirmation. I wasn't exactly going to pop out my own teeth and give them a scrub mid-shift, was I? What did she take me for?

In the end, Sandy had a beautiful baby born via forceps in the theatre. Thankfully her teeth remained in situ for the birth, and no one would ever have known. In a way I was pleased it was forceps as I didn't have enough hands to stand by to catch her teeth and let alone her baby. Once we warded Sandy and her baby, Diane and I were walking back to Delivery Suite, and she started laughing.

'What's the matter?' I said smiling intrigued for what she was about to say.

Sorry Meg, I just can't believe you cleaned someone's teeth today. Whilst they weren't even in her mouth,' she sniggered. I felt a hand on my back and turned to see Helen standing with her scrub hat half off her head.

'Students do pretty much anything for vaginal births but Meg, a patient's top set of teeth? That's a new one,' Helen said and walked away smiling to herself. Brilliant. But, honestly, if cleaning dislodged teeth meant I got to facilitate a vaginal birth, I'd do it all again tomorrow. Maybe with a mouth guard next time.

CHAPTER
Fifty

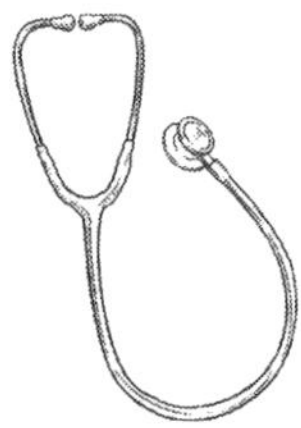

WHY IS IT ALWAYS ME?

Another January, another birthday and another excuse for a trip to the Celtic Manor. Bea and I finished our last lecture on Friday the seventh and headed straight for South Wales. I always loved the drive and how when the panorama of rolling hills came into focus, I knew home was close. Bea and I had a few questionable looks from other drivers as she fist pumped the air and I shimmied my shoulders to the beat of Mcfly as we Mcflew across the motorway as it were.

Eventually pulling up to the Celtic Manor I felt like my birthday was really getting started; I was wearing my special-occasion lengthy coat which made me feel like someone important from London or something, so I knew it was a special occasion when I whipped it out of the wardrobe. Excitedly, I got out almost instantly and watched my little red Toyota roll slowly down the hill realising I'd clearly not put the handbrake on well enough. Bollocks! My heart fell through my arse as I abandoned my bags and scrambled down the incline. Bea said it looked like my coat took flight before I did, like a superhero in a minor-key Marvel spinoff: Super Meg or The Incompetent Avenger? Although what she didn't see was how I hung onto the wing mirror, flung the door open and desperately pulled myself in and yanked my handbrake up as far it could go. Not so Super Meg.

'Thank God for that,' I huffed which steamed up my glasses which had been dislodged further down my face. I was moments away from a sand bunker so thought I'd better get myself out of this asap.

'Alright there Meg?' A red-faced Bea said laughing so much I thought she may keel over from lack of oxygen at any moment.

'All is in hand,' I shoved my thumbs up and my feet to it seemed; with again no handbrake and no pressure on the brake now, my car jolted forward in a state of engine cease.

'Yes, I fucking stalled', I said seriously which lasted approximately a second then both I and Bea were sharing hysterics. A brilliant start.

When I'd actually driven the car back to the designated space and lifted the handbrake up to the Gods above, I deemed it safe to leave and headed for the hotel. The hotel sat fetching on top of the blunt-edged grass. Flawlessly trimmed trees stood tall around the entrance and were flecked with lights from the festive period. However, due to us being a little bit later than last year, there was a ladder against one of the trees with a man at the top collecting the never-ending string of lights. He looked like a little spec compared to the trees he was faced with. God help him if he fell in, I don't think we'd see him on this side of the year. Anyway, hoping that man was going to make it through January with the rest of us, we checked in and headed for our room. Just like last time, our room was faultless and elegant, everything I was not.

After settling in, we prepped for the spa; I grinned at our white-robed reflections, and we made a beeline for the bottom floor. I couldn't wait to just let my mind drift onto anything but midwifery, essays, lectures, and placement. I was after some inner peace to carry into my twenty-second year, as after all it had been a topsy-turvy twenty-two years. This was quickly disrupted when the lift binged, and we entered with people dressed in formal attire without a hair out of place. I just looked like a bald eyebrowed, hair slicked back into a bun on the top of my head, no bra so boobs swept the floor more than Cinderella ever did kind of girl. I embarrassedly smiled at the people who had paused their conversation to scan me. Bea, on the other hand, was trying not to laugh, I shared the humour once we were firmly away from the prestigious group.

'That was not okay!' I exclaimed rubbing my eyebrows as if they were going to appear after three rubs like The Genie. Without the appearance of Genie eyebrows, Bea dragged me over to the check-in desk and we headed for the changing rooms.

Thankfully, no formal wear was in sight and everyone else was also pool-ready, so we blended in seamlessly. I did fifteen lengths of the dimly lit pool, finding every stroke through the turquoise water a calming force. Bea did a couple with me and retired to the hot tub. An elite choice. I finally joined her, and we reflected on life as it was, people, placement, the funny, and the ugly, we put the world to rights from a tiny corner of it. Eventually, we got out and headed for the sauna. I couldn't cope for long and felt like my bronchioles were catching alight. Like a dry forest fire, I felt the heat spread across my chest. I panicked and moved rapidly towards the exit. Gasping for a few breaths of now seemingly icy cold air I had a few people ask me if I was okay to which I told them I had a cheeky bit of asthma rather than revealing the truth of my inability to cope with hot air. Although Bea said she was the same and came out shortly after me. We decided to go to the steam room next, with the hope that the water wouldn't make me sound like I had a continuous dry cough, which was the code for Covid these days.

I could barely see through the clouds of vapour in front of me when we entered the steam room. I don't know what I was expecting to be fair but, I held my arms out in front of me and led myself to the bench. I then realised it was a little rectangular room without a great deal of space actually, compared to the other rooms in the vicinity. There was a man to my right and Bea tapped me and pointed at a man to her left, someone we must have passed on the way in but didn't see. Anyway, we spent the first five minutes eyes closed and listening to the soft trickles of water droplets around us. I only opened them when the mystery man on the left exited.

I wondered how long he managed. Anyway, the other silhouette of the man on my right came into clearer focus as he shuffled across the bench toward me. I subtly analysed his features and found him to look about sixty-something and in a fair physical state with only a small protruding stomach edging its way over his shorts. I dreaded to think of myself in my sixties based on my current physique.

'Alright?' He said to me as we caught each other's glance. I gave him a thumbs-up and a smile. Something stopped me from talking, which was inconsistent with me. Bea opened her eyes and turned to assess the situation as she too thought it odd that she didn't hear me reply.

'Lovely this is init?' He said trying Bea now. 'Hitting the spot real good', he said as he repositioned himself, again closer to me which I shuffled a space closer to Bea. He seemed to get the hint and left us to close our eyes again. Although I was on alert to him to be fair and would only truly relax when he'd gone. There was just something about him that made me feel uneasy.

A few minutes went by, and I heard a few slaps on the wet tiles. Thankful it was him leaving as I hadn't heard the door go for someone to come in, I reshuffled my shoulders and leaned them back into the wall. But the slaps continued. I instinctively opened my eyes and regardless of my bald eyebrows, my expression was in obvious shock. I stared in horror as he began... planking. No, thrusting. Plusthing? It was origin of the slapping noise that disturbed me the most. He lowered his stomach and pelvis to the floor over and over and over again. I gave Bea a strong nudge and her face was a picture. Again, unsure of how to react to a pre-pensioner thrusting on the steam room floor, she sat in a state of shock also.

'Yeah, woo, this is how you stay well every day,' he announced mid-thrust which startled both Bea and I into a jump. Why did he have to do it now of all time? Somehow, I bet he wouldn't have done it whilst the Mystery guy on the left was in there...

'Hard work this, but it keeps me clean', he said although we definitely did not ask. I started to smirk eventually, perplexed at what I was actually witnessing. Bea on the other hand grabbed my wrist as she fled for the door. We both hurried over to the empty hot tub, almost dived in there and hid ourselves underneath bubbles.

'No, it's actually not funny', Bea said wiping bubbles off of her head. 'What on earth was he doing? That was disgusting', she deduced.

'I have no idea, I'm gonna say he was working out as the alternative, ugh, I dread to think about it', I shivered and flung a few bubbles sideways. 'Why is it always us?' I asked her, laughing now.

'Woah Meg, why is it always *you?* No man has ever thrust his pelvis to the ground at me before!' She laughed at the consistent magnetism I had for bizarre situations. It looked like twenty-two wasn't going to be any different after all; cars rolling down hills, looking like the biggest anomaly amongst formal attire in my dressing gown and witnessing a half-naked sixty-plus-year-old repeatedly plunge himself into the floor and peel himself back off it.

'Happy twenty-second, Meg,' Bea cheered a particularly wet cardboard cup of water my way. I crossed my eyes in response anticipating another year of utter carnage.

CHAPTER
Fifty-One

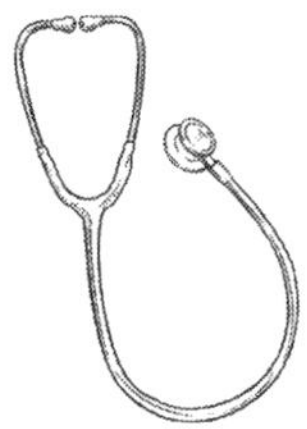

REMEMBRANCE

Even in a world where we often find a little sun between the clouds, sometimes the sky just stays grey. As we all know, death is an inevitable consequence of living. Nevertheless, when a person dies, for those of us who loved them, we feel that painful grief which hurts a devastating physical pain, which someone told me once, essentially sits where love lived before. Although midwifery is predominantly a positive time for a lot of families, there are of course devastating circumstances, when a baby dies. Knowing they had their whole life ahead of them, we reflect on what their first word would have been, their hair colour, their personality, and who they would have grown up to be. For that to disappear, is simply shattering. Whether a baby is lost at ten, twenty, thirty, or forty weeks, the grief remains the same. Age doesn't measure love.

I remember all of the babies who have died that I have had the privilege to care for. I remember their families and what I did for each of them. It's something that sticks with you given the heartbreaking importance of the care they need. The first baby I ever cared for who died was called Poppy. It was November, the month of remembrance. I'd pinned a red poppy to my lanyard, unaware at the time how poignant that would become. When her mum saw it, she paused.

'That's her name,' she said. We talked for a while, just about Poppy. Her name. It was the first time I saw her smile in two days. That little poppy has been there ever since.

CHAPTER

Fifty-Two

TWO BABIES, ONE PROPOSAL AND NO TIME LEFT IN THE DAY

PART ONE

A few days after caring for Poppy and her family, I returned to Delivery Suite to find they were no longer there. I guess it was crazy how things changed so rapidly in that environment. I was working with a midwife called Alice this time, who was pleasant enough for me to have a go at leading, knowing she would help if needed.

Sadia, para nought, thirty-nine weeks, no adverse medical history, but on Delivery Suite due to being induced for recurrent reduced fetal movements. Upon introduction to Sadia and her family, they told me that Sadia's partner was in another country and her dad who was standing in instead, happened to be a consultant anesthetist, so the pressure was on. I almost vommed when I found out. Her mum was a dentist, so I felt slightly more relaxed in that sense.

'What happens if I don't progress?' Sadia asked worriedly as she examined the syringe of oxytocin that was keeping her contracting well. I explained our options, and Alice nodded in the background, which felt like a moment to be proud of.

'She could have an epidural top-up if we go to the theatre,' Rajan, Sadia's dad, deduced as he examined the epidural pump. 'Who's the anesthetist on the call today, please?' he asked curiously. I had no idea, so I turned to Alice for that one.

'I believe it's Anthony,' she said thoughtfully.

'Is he good, Dad?' Sadia asked with her big brown eyes, looking deep into his for an honest answer.

'He's good, but he is not yet consultant. Can I not come into the theatre?' he looked towards me, again the one without the full answer on this.

'Only one other person is allowed in the theatre with Sadia if theatre is needed, but I think you're doing an excellent job', I turned to Sadia, 'You and your body are doing exactly what we would want at the present time,' I tried to reassure them and change the subject simultaneously. Still, Rajan swished his hand back and forth, a silencing signal which did cause a minor feeling of offence come to the surface. Thankfully, Alice stepped in and bluntly reiterated that he wouldn't usually be able to join as Sadia had already elected her mum, and especially not in an anesthetic capacity as this was his daughter also.

A couple of hours passed, and on the subsequent examination, Sadia's cervix remained at six centimetres but appeared to have gotten swollen. The baby's head didn't feel it was in an optimal position either. We were querying obstruction (of labour) at this stage as Sadia stopped being able to pass urine, too, a classic red flag. One of our doctors reviewed and was in the middle of explaining her options when, all of a sudden, the baby's heart rate hit eighty bpm and lasted long enough to deem it a fetal bradycardia. Emergency bells were hit, and the team summoned instantly. Rajan leapt to his feet and started combing down his hair in the reflection of the epidural box in preparation for something. Although it was unclear what a new hairdo would provide, I wasn't sure how Anthony would take Rajan as he was not on duty.

Anthony was incredibly confident with his practice but also very autonomous, preferring to work solo wherever possible. He had a polished, bald head, which he would perch his theatre hat on the top of, and he wore his theatre gown open so when he took significant strides down the corridor, his literal cape would ripple in the air behind him. He was like a super-anesthetist. He's even been seen to habitually wink at midwives and flex his solid upper torso. He told us once that he goes to the gym four times a week, so there was no wonder his biceps had biceps. He behaved and looked legitimately like Gaston from Beauty and the Beast, but with slightly better manners. But that was Anthony for you, and again, I couldn't foreknow how he would respond to Rajan.

Thankfully, the baby's heart rate recovered when we changed Sadia's position. Our obstetric registrar found her to be six centimetres and oedematous still. So, given fetal distress and that the baby was continuing to decelerate following the bradycardia, the decision was for a caesarean section.

'That's fine with me; I'm quite happy to be comfortable now and have him out whichever way,' Sadia said casually.

The theatre team was called to congregate in our room and get her prepped alongside me. Who was first up to arrive? Anthony. He gave a firm, wholehearted knock and swung the door open. He almost lunged into the room with his cloak gliding behind him.

'I am Anthony,' he announced proudly, 'I am your anesthetist,' he broadened his shoulders. As much as I commended him for his work and fully supported him to be proud of himself, I couldn't ignore that he had just watched another deep deceleration but kept smiling his pearly whites at her. At least Sadia's mum would be impressed. Although, I needed him to kindly get out of his arse and come back down to earth.

'Rajan,' Oh, here we go. 'Consultant anesthetist, a pleasure to meet you, Anthony. Can you tell me your plans for top-up or spinal?' Again, asking whilst the baby's CTG was deteriorating, and we needed to get a move on. It was a standoff between the anesthetists where I felt like I was on Gladiators; in the blue corner, a renowned anesthetic consultant who has worked in over ten countries in the last decade, his reputation...exceptional. In the red corner is none other than our existing anesthetist; he has both the physical and mental strength of an ox... indestructible. Who will come out on top? I was keen to find out, but equally, that CTG was getting worse, so I left the room to get my parts of the preparation for theatre to speed up the process. By the time I returned, Anthony was deep in conversation with Natalie, the only band seven I'd met so far who didn't have the personality of a stale custard cream. Meanwhile, Rajan was brandishing his NHS badge like a backstage pass at Glastonbury.

'Okay, so, Sadia, I've got you an antacid here, and I just need to run through this checklist before we head in,' I said with Alice behind me.

'I'm not ready yet, Megan,' she said calmly as she fiddled with the bag on her bedside.

'We need to go as soon as we can, Sadia; your baby is distressed,' I tried to be both clear and sensitive.

'I'd like to do my makeup before,' she said as she got out her mirror and foundation.

'No, as in your baby is distressed and needs to be born now,' Alice supported me.

'No, I've made a choice that the team can wait for a few minutes,' she concluded. I was quite taken aback that she was applying full-on makeup while her baby was hanging on. Maybe she didn't quite understand the urgency, as we were all clearly too good at being calm in an emergency. Alice and I reiterated that the baby was distressed and needed out. However, she continued to decline and requested we inform the team.

'This will *not* go down well,' Alice turned to me, the colour draining slowly from her face. Alice knocked on the office door and we said a prayer anticipating being crucified.

We explained all to Jane and the rest of the room as naturally, they were all listening to the gossip.

'Sorry?' Jane asked perplexed.

'She's literally declined,' Alice confirmed, 'I can't force her to go against her will.'

'We've been through it all, multiple times too,' I added. Jane swiveled on her chair to face the multi view screen for CTGs.

'Fucks sake,' she said as she bumped her head on the desk beneath her.

'Well, that didn't go well did it,' Alice turned to me as we left the office back to Sadia's room. I've never hoped to see someone with her eyebrows on so much as I did in that moment. Thankfully, eyebrows, mascara were indeed on, and she was on the last bits. Eventually, we got Sadia to the theatre with her gown on and her whole face of makeup up, of course. She even put on eyelashes, which was nothing other than impressive at that point, to be honest. Mind you, they were twice the length they were half an hour ago; our theatre nurse squinted when she saw us approaching, and I couldn't help but think that she probably saw Sadia's eyelashes before her.

Theatre was interesting, to say the least; Rajan had been given a compromise by Jane and stood at the back of the theatre, but Anthony, on the other hand, kept throwing Rajan disapproving looks, clearly not impressed he was being observed. Meanwhile, when Sadia had her spinal, she had a vasovagal episode and fainted. Brilliant. We had to reposition her, her dad was barking orders at the back of theatre (another reason why more than one family member generally don't come in, let alone when you're an anesthetist too).

During the commotion of us stabilising Sadia, her eyelashes started to unstick as the glue wasn't quite dry yet. They were then swept from her real eyelashes by her own involuntary hand movements across her face, which she kept doing.

Ultimately, we had a distressed baby, two anesthetists firing each other looks as they turned the theatre into a battlefield, and Sadia's eyelashes were malting. It was like confetti; a couple were now glued to the sides of her face and looked like overly asymmetrical sideburns.

We even found a few later outside of her catheter tube. I will never know how they managed to get there. The highlight of this was that, in recovery, Sadia asked me earnestly if her pubic hair had started falling out as a result of her spinal, imagine writing, 'Query spinal-induced pubic alopecia' in her notes. I barely held it together when I confirmed they were her eyelashes and that her pubes were intact. She was mortified when she looked in the mirror and found herself looking like a makeshift Elvis with bits of hair everywhere and very uneven eyelashes. Oh, and last but not least, thankfully our distressed baby came out healthy and crying, in the best condition of all that went to theatre in that group.

PART TWO

LATER THAT DAY, ALICE AND I HAD TO TAKE A LABOURing multip from triage. I felt the tingles of excitement make their way around my body. I was on thirty-three spontaneous vaginal births facilitated at this point, eighty-two percent towards the qualifying goal of forty, so I was undoubtedly getting there now. Alice and I entered room three, where we found Ashleigh sitting on the bed as her triage midwife strapped her to the CTG. Alice introduced herself, and when I opened my mouth to introduce myself, Ashleigh became very vocal with her next contraction. I exchanged an enthusiastic look with Alice as we thought the same thing; a particular sound a woman makes sounds like advanced labour. I can't describe it, but I can now understand where someone is based on their sound. Of course, one rule doesn't fit all, and someone once was incredibly silent, and in the end, her baby delivered itself without us having much of a clue, but that is a story for another time. For Ashleigh, the depth of her voice during a contraction alighted with the pressure she felt, and as we had predicted, she powered herself through labour, and her baby subsequently got lower and lower into her pelvis. Thankfully, her partner, Mike, arrived at about seven centimeters quickly after sorting their other three kids at different places.

'Bloody hell, Ash, you don't half do it quick,' was the first thing he said to her upon his arrival.

'Ahh, love, I'm so glad you made it,' she exhaled with pure relief. Alice gestured for Mike to stash the bags in the bathroom.

'Burly work, hey,' he rubbed his hands together.

'You're telling me,' Ashleigh said as she gestured for him to go over to her. 'Jesus Christ,' she clamored as her abdomen visibly hardened with the next contraction.

'No gas and air yet, then, babe?' He looked surprised. Ashleigh shook her head as she shuddered off the last of that contraction. 'She usually asks for it about ten minutes before they come out,' he said, shining with pride. I remember enjoying the love and appreciation they had for each other. That's one thing I miss about being a student; since being qualified, the responsibility shot through the roof, and the clinical need supersedes the rest (in your head). Although my exterior image encourages all sentimental things, they register in your brain as great as the experience is clearly going well for the family. Still, you instantly move back to monitoring the CTG, infusions and whatever else. Being a student, you are protected from that liability and can be still and truly in that moment occasionally. I found I was only ever emotional during a birth during my training. Have I become cold-hearted? No, I've become hardened by responsibility and accountability. But from the outside, I'm the same as I've always been, and that's all that matters to our patient body.

Ashleigh was chatting between her contractions, which always gave us a false sense of security. She and Mike told us their life story so far; three kids and twenty years of being together. They met in a hospital, visiting elderly family members at the time. They always said having their babies felt like full circle moments, and for them, their happiest times had only ever been in hospitals. They were the rarity that liked to be in that environment, and I'm sure half of us would love to feel the same.

'Mikey, I can't hack this anymore,' Ashleigh said as she grabbed his shoulders.

Mike flicked his eyebrows up and down in mine and Alice's direction, and we all knew what was next. Ashleigh looked longingly into Mike's eyes until he wiped away a tear and said, 'It's time,' like a pivotal point in a movie. And in all fairness, it was a pivotal point in theirs as not even a minute after we gave her entonox, Ashleigh started uncontrollably pushing. Lots of water gushed out each time, an obvious symptom of unbearable pressure and descent. After a few pushes, Ashleigh wanted to lie on the bed. We encouraged her that she didn't have to be on the bed for the baby to be born, as many of us assume; however, Mike said this is how she did it every time. Fair enough. He helped her onto the bed, and the baby's head started edging its way out. I coached Ashleigh whilst Alice called for our second midwife, who prepared the syntometrine and wrote times on the CTG.

'Go on, Ash, go on, love!' Mike kissed her hand, which was tightly grasping his. One hearty push and baby's head birthed into my hands.

'Brilliant, Ashleigh, on the next contr-'Ashleigh had already started pushing again, 'Now is as good a time as any; you've got this!' Their baby entered the world in one swift motion: shoulders, body, feet and a complete little boy wearing vernix, blood and a cross face, fuming he'd been evicted from his lovely, warm abode.

'Congratulations both, Ashleigh. You did brilliantly,' I said as I lifted him to his Mum for the first time. Ashleigh seized him with both hands and placed him on her chest. Mike leaned over them, emotion pouring out of his eyes.

'You're crying on him, love,' Ashleigh laughed as another big droplet splashed onto their little man's shoulders. I replaced the pads under Ashleigh as the originals were soaked with the elements of birth. When I turned around from the bin, Mike wasn't anywhere to be seen, and Ashleigh was peering over her bedside. Oh god, he surely can't have fainted, can he?

'Four births, and now he faints!' Ashleigh chuckled. 'That's the first time he's done that!' she said as Alice made a beeline to Mike to confirm his well-being. It turned out he was, in fact, on the floor, not unconscious, but on one knee.

'Ash,' Mike started.

'You alright, love?' She called out to the air, not able to see him over her legs, which were suspended into lithotomy as Ashleigh had requested, so she wasn't touching her blood; she said she had a weird thing about it after her babies were born. Again, fair enough.

'Twenty wonderful years,' Mike went on, still Ashleigh couldn't see him.

'Oh my god, are you proposing?' Ashleigh caught on eventually, although in all fairness, she had just pushed a baby out. 'Is he proposing?' Ashleigh mouthed to me. Mike went on to pour his heart out to his partner, who was suspended several feet in the air, legs spread apart after a baby had just come out of her vagina, who still couldn't see him. I got onto the bed control panel and started edging Ashleigh down so they could at least see each other, although this particular bed kept stopping and starting. Typical.'You are the light of all of our lives.' JOLT. 'The kids adore you, and I couldn't be prouder.' JOLT. 'So, after all of our happy times in hospitals...' JOLT. 'Will you marry me?'

'Oh my god, yes, Mikey, yes!' Ashleigh squealed. Mike jumped up and gave her the amplest hug.

'Plus, I'm getting the snip after this one, so this is likely our last happy trip to a hospital; I thought we'd have to go out with a baby and a ring,' he beamed as he revealed a sparkling diamond. Ashleigh put her hands over her mouth, letting go of her baby. Alice had to push him back to the centre; the poor guy got wedged between her boobs.

'Shall we cut baby's cord now?' I asked, and Mike and Ashleigh turned to me as if they had forgotten I was still there. 'It's stopped pulsating now, so all of that extra blood will have gotten to baby now?' I said to their blank faces.

'I guess that's another thing I'll say yes to today,' Ashleigh beamed.

Later that night, I went to fill up my car with petrol en route home. The guy at the station saw me looking tired and asked how my day was. Was it appropriate to say that someone thought her eyelashes were pubes, and another technically asked someone's vagina to marry him as he couldn't see her face? I went for a 'nice, thank you' in the end as most of us would.

CHAPTER
Fifty-Three

DISS-ENGAGING - I'M BUSY

Following baby thirty-four and witnessing a proposal, we returned to theory block where our lecturers spoke the unspoken word. The dreaded dissertation. A critical submission launched in most people's final year of university. The objective of 10,000 words felt more like 10,000 hours. What did that even equate to in real time? According to Google: 417 days. Honestly, that felt generous. It devoured my time more than anything else; mostly because I would go on a tangent, re-read it and realise it wasn't even relevant and end up deleting it all. Back to square one often meant a cry into my paper coffee cup at the student union, marking life at its finest.

What always made me laugh was that the word 'dissertation' in itself, held so much weight with out any context. Just mention 'the diss' and you're excused. If you need to get out of something all you just had to mention was the magic word. I remember a group of friends asking if I wanted to go out clubbing and considering my past experiences, my answer was a firm no. Although my justification of 'sorry its just not my scene', wasn't a good enough answer for them so they continued to push me for ages to come. In the end, I mentioned 'the diss' and that was it, they dropped it instantly. I was mesmerised and started embracing my newfound ally.

1. 'Can you come to the ward meeting to represent the student midwives?'

'So sorry, I'm drowning in the diss,' I'd say back as sadly as I could muster.

2. 'Coming shopping, Meg?'

'No sorry, bashing the diss out!' *She swipes on Farm Heroes*

3. 'Midwifery social?'

'Dissertation, sorry.'

'But Meg, we submitted it last week?' *Fuck.*

In all fairness, before that last time when it was past the submission date, I didn't really have time for anything other than study. Bea and I spent the month leading up to its submission in our sacred place of work, leisure, general make-life-better place, Starbucks. My acknowledgements should have mentioned the iconic caffeine filled phenomenon and how I may as well have set up a direct debit to them seen as I spent most of my student finance (and now wage) there; at least three different baristas knew my name, order and how many words I'd written each time.

Only twenty-one days after submitting it and the results were in. I passed! With the academic side of the degree complete, I reflected on how I found my imposter syndrome was beginning to lessen. It was a sacred thing to experience and a moment when like all have said before me, the light at the end of the tunnel appeared. Although gutted I couldn't excuse myself from absolutely everything anymore, I was thrilled to have passed it. Again, I missed the diss in a very toxic relationship kind of way. But onwards. Eight weeks of clinical placement. Six more babies. And then, I could finally qualify as a midwife. And leave shitty X behind, forever.

CHAPTER *Fifty-Four*

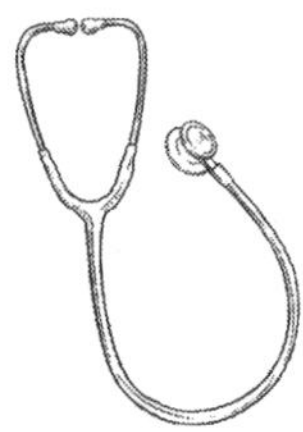

THE STOCKROOM HAS EYES

Another lesson I learned the hard way, on one of those Delivery Suite shifts where your mentor hates you, and you end up hating yourself even more. We had a patient have an emergency caesarean section as soon as we started, followed by two elective caesarean sections that were not as straight forward as anticipated.

One lost over a litre of blood and crashed into hypotension. The other went the opposite way; her blood pressure was so high we were practically peeling the readings off the ceiling. The mentor I was working with wasn't the worst I'd worked with, not by far. However, she made it clear she didn't want to be in work that day and made me feel uneasy too many times to recall. The final straw was when I was asked by a different midwife to help her for a minute as she was so busy. My mentor was in the staffroom as we didn't have a patient at this time, so I completed a few tasks for her which took me about twenty minutes. On my return, my mentor stood up and asked me where the hell I'd been? Despite my explanation of helping out another colleague, she told me off for 'absconding' and not asking permission to do something else, which hit me in the pit of my stomach. I felt a rise in anger from my stomach up to my chest which saw me flee to the stockroom. I was so pissed off and felt if I didn't move then I may have given her something to tell me off for...

I stormed off into the kitchen stockroom and as soon as the door closed, I shot my two middle fingers in front of me bringing them back and forth to say a big fuck off. I spun around and flailed my arms up with all the pent-up energy I'd been holding back. I was pretty done, can you tell? I was just sick and tired of the constant bad vibes.

A couple of nights later when I was chatting with the other girls in the house, one of the girls mentioned a really embarrassing story about how one of the consultants at X got caught stealing patient orange juice cartons from the stock cupboard the other day and the midwives were all watching the replay on the cameras. My face dropped like a sad, half-deflated party balloon. Cameras. Caught. Embarrassing. My brain started doing backflips. I started freaking out slightly and excused myself from the others. A few minutes later Bea arrived.

'Meg, what's the matter?' she asked, stepping into my room.

'I gave the stockroom door both middle fingers and some... interpretative rage dancing.' Her mouth twitched.

'Nooo...' she said trying her level best to conceal a smile.

'What if they watch that back?' I groaned, smothering my face with both hands like that would now somehow protect my identity.

'Nah, don't worry,' she said, still clearly enjoying this. 'They probably only check footage if something goes missing. You're safe.' I flopped back dramatically.

'God whyyyyy.' If I didn't already have one foot out of X, that CCTV footage had just given me the final shove.

CHAPTER *Fifty-Five*

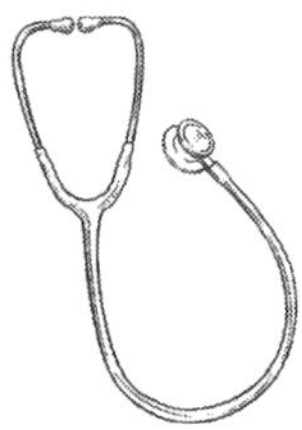

THE PENULTIMATE CHAPTER

Babies thirty-nine and forty came into the world on yet another overtime shift I had to do, but this time, it was the shift that marked the end of my training. I couldn't believe I'd made it, through the devastation, humiliation, and the kind of oppression that creeps in slowly until you forget what it's like to breathe properly. Nobody seemed to care that it was my last day apart from the wonderful mentor that I did have that last shift, if only there were more of her. Nevertheless, I remember throwing my hands up to the hospital and whooping as I flew out of the doors. I had a few looks that questioned my seemingly unprovoked happiness, from other members of staff and the public. My grin just got wider. X's maternity services wouldn't be getting another ounce of my time, my kindness or me. Ha! The taste of freedom was almost as good as a strawberry ice cream, the closest contender in a long time.

So, to those who made my life hell, this grin's for you. May you never meet anyone like yourselves. And if you do:

1. Stay hydrated. Tears don't make themselves.
2. Don't drive depressed, it is a new edition of the 'don't drive drunk' lesson, but specific to how people like you make some of us feel instead of alcohol.
3. Budget for breakdowns. That's £120 a year on antidepressants, £120 on anti-anxiety meds, and God knows how much on private therapy. It's essential, and extortionate.
4. And finally: the good always wins. Maybe not today. Maybe not next week. But it does. It really, really does.

CHAPTER Fifty-Six

QUALIFIED FREEDOM

I've always been partial to a silver lining, or a thousand of them. And over the last three years, I've had no shortage of reasons to smile: from synonyms for vagina to rogue dentures on Delivery Suite. Laughing was, and still is, one of the best things humans can share, right up there with love, loyalty, and the kind of kindness that doesn't ask for anything back.

To the soul-bright midwives of X who kept me going, thank you. For believing in me when I didn't, for offering shelter in a storm I couldn't explain, and for showing that goodness can exist even in a system that too often forgets it. I sound like I'm giving a BAFTA speech, don't I? Honestly, after what we've all been through, I think we deserved one.

Cheers to all of the student midwives out there, this isn't an easy gig. Though I guess the official prize was the degree, and the NMC pin, right? Plot twist, we paid £28,500 for, which is somehow more than a midwife's starting salary. Brilliant.

Still, I didn't just graduate with a BSc. I came out with a few extra letters too: PTSD/A+D. Stick that on a CV and it looks like I'm a professor in psychological warfare. But none of those letters mean as much as the people behind them. So, to the real heroes of this story, my family and friends, thank you. For the late-night calls, the pep talks, the unconditional love, the patience, the 'you're not actually crap at this' reminders and the belief that never once faltered. Thank you for always being team Meg. You were the reason I made it through. I love you more than I could ever write down. This qualification might have my name on it, but it belongs to all of us. So, I accept this award of qualified freedom with a full heart, singed nerves, and the steady hands you helped build.

Now let's see what happens when Hurricane Meg hits the world of midwifery. All it takes is a different coloured dress, a qualified pin...

...and maybe, just maybe, enough content for a second memoir. Stay tuned.

Printed in Dunstable, United Kingdom

81719056R00205